Awakening to Wholeness

A LIFE UNMASKED

BY
Rochelle Trow

ISBN: 979-8-89669-028-3

DEDICATION

To my beloved twin boys,

In the beautiful chaos of motherhood, you have been my greatest teacher. Your laughter has brightened my darkest days, and your unique spirits have shown me the true meaning of love, patience, and resilience. This journey has not always been easy; it has been filled with challenges that tested my strength and vulnerability. Yet, I have learned through every struggle that our bond deepens through openness, understanding, and acceptance.

May this book serve as a testament to the love that binds us—a love that thrives in the freedom to grow, explore, and embrace our individuality. Thank you for allowing me to be your mother and teaching me that the heart of family lies in compassion and connection. Together, we will continue to navigate this beautiful adventure of life, hand in hand, heart to heart.

Endorsements for Awakening to Wholeness: A Life Unmasked

This book is a gift for anyone seeking clarity, resilience, and the freedom to embrace their truest self.

As both an executive coach and author, I have had the privilege of witnessing Rochelle's transformative journey firsthand. In "Awakening to Wholeness: a Life Unmasked," she offers a deeply authentic and masterfully written memoir that transcends personal storytelling to touch on universal truths about leadership, resilience, and authenticity.

Rochelle's reflections reveal a leader's courage to confront hard truths, honour her roots, and embrace freedom—all while maintaining clarity, compassion, and self-awareness. Her journey from corporate shadows to clarity is particularly inspiring, as it demonstrates the power of aligning one's inner and outer life to lead with purpose and integrity.

This book is a testament to the transformational journey every great leader must undertake—moving beyond roles and expectations to uncover their true essence. Rochelle's authenticity and remarkable maturity make her story compelling and a valuable guide for leaders seeking to inspire others by first leading themselves. This remarkable work is a must-read for anyone ready to awaken to their wholeness and elevate their leadership.

Nicole Heimann: Award Winning CEO Coach

Author "How to Develop the Authentic Leader in You"

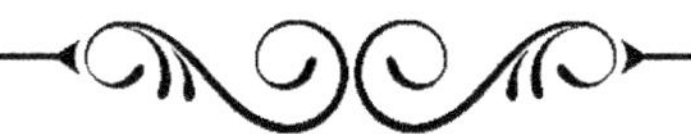

This book is an invitation, a call to be brave - for you. To answer the timeless call to "know thyself", to hear and trust the answers within you.

As an executive coach and former HR leader, I have seen what it means to go along to get along in the corporate world. Along the way, you lose who you truly are, piece by piece, trying to live up to the demands and expectations of everyone around you. This is an invitation to those leaders, to courageously step into your authenticity. It's a big invitation, I know! But Rochelle shows us how she is like a guide walking alongside you, using her story to guide you in rewriting your own. She shows us we have the power inside ourselves to write a new story.

Rochelle vulnerably shares stories of her origin family, sharing what she had to do to receive love as a child. These personal stories illuminate how our early relationships create a relationship blueprint for how we lead, how we engage others, how we deal with challenges, conflicts and the unknown. She shows leaders how to invite stillness and become more self-aware and in doing so, to confront their light and shadow sides, with grace and self-compassion and in doing so to unlock something new.

She shows mothers and women how to peel back the masks, break out of the moulds, shed the labels and roles we take on and break away from repeating the same patterns and cycles of behaviour that keep us trapped. She shows families that we can honour our roots and ancestry and with acceptance and forgiveness we can heal generational trauma with the understanding that our parents did their best, so we can do better for our children. She shows that sisterhood and friendship is a powerful means of support and in a world that is becoming lonelier, that to develop meaningful connections is an intentional act, that starts with you. She shows that the journey back to your true essence can take many forms and yet there is a clear message of being open and present to what arises, to do less and to be more.

From apartheid South Africa to the calm tranquility of Switzerland, Rochelle illustrates the wisdom of Ubuntu, that we are all interconnected, that people are only people through other people. That we cannot and should not do this life alone. It takes a village to grow as humans. I am the eldest grandchild she writes about who made her an aunt at 5 years old, but to me, Rochelle has always been my big sister. Always present and supportive in my life, it's an honour and inspiration to watch her grow and to see her free herself and use her voice to help others find theirs.

Awakening to Wholeness: A Life Unmasked, is an invitation to love and accept yourself for who you truly are.

Melanie Peck, The Journey Coach

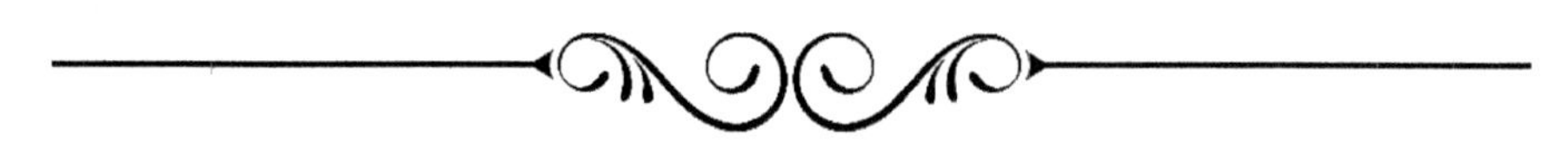

What if you achieved everything you thought you wanted - only to find you're still not happy?

It is a fascinating journey of self-reflection, insight and discovery. Rochelle shares her personal story with a transparency and rawness that is inspiring, relatable and real. Her tale will have you alternately gasping in shock and cheering with joy. Her journey is an example of facing fears, letting go of pain, discovering what truly matters on the path to more meaningful relationships and a genuinely fulfilling life.

Rochelle's reflections cover the full range of wellness, including insights and implications for improving mind, body and soul. Her experience illuminates the benefits of investing in yourself, believing in yourself and the intrinsic value of mental wellbeing as a doorway to healing and self-discovery. While everyone's journey is different, Rochelle offers clear insights she has gained through this experience. She provides the reader with practical nuggets of how to develop our minds, cultivate inner peace, rediscover love, and honestly know ourselves.

Adam Zaeske, Healthcare Executive

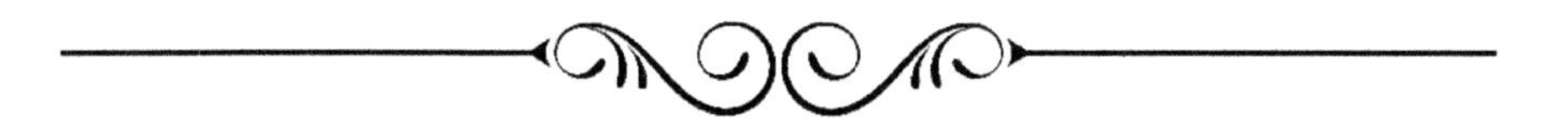

A guide to becoming who you were always meant to be.

Given Rochelle's start in life, she truly exemplifies the expression, "self-made". We met as colleagues at the start of our careers, and I was inspired by the tenacious way in which she earned her seat at the top table of the global leadership teams of major international organisations. A South African woman of colour, she commanded respect in the corporate world before movements like "Black Lives Matter" and "Me-too" helped to make workplaces more accepting of difference. Rochelle herself was a driving force behind culture change in the workplace we shared – and beyond. It was both astonishing and brave that she then set off on a different path - a difficult and sometimes painful journey to her true self. She transformed her life based on her essence, vision, purpose, and her own definition of success.

In *Awakening to Wholeness: a Life Unmasked,* Rochelle tells her unique story with unflinching honesty and generously shares the lessons she learned along the way. Her words resonate with the same wisdom and compassion that have guided her clients, myself included. She has been an unwavering source of strength and support when I needed it most, in both my professional career and personal life, for which I will always be thankful.

Awakening to Wholeness is much more than Rochelle's inspiring story - her reflections offer a guide to finding and radiating your inner light. The book will be particularly helpful to those who are ready to embark on their own journeys of self-discovery.

Bonita Dordel, Communications Director and friend who has become family

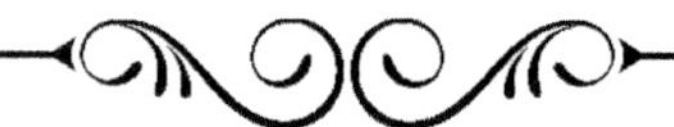

Awakening to Wholeness: A Life Unmasked is a book truly defined by its title.

I've learnt so much about my heritage and insights into my father's side of the family post being estranged for many years. It helps me understand the initial disconnection and makes me appreciate the reconnection so much more, despite the difficult circumstances under which this took place. Reading the book, I feel grateful for Rochelle. Not only for the impactful role that she has played in my life for over 20 years but the vulnerability and authenticity that she has poured out on each page. Sharing the highs, lows, and hidden "raw" parts of herself will open the hearts and minds of every reader to reflect on their own lives, and we will undoubtedly be better off doing it! In Marianne Williamson's words, *"Our deepest fear is not that we are inadequate. Our deepest fear is that we are powerful beyond measure. It is our light, not our darkness that most frightens us."* May this book encourage readers to ask "Who am I truly?". May it become the stepping stone for change, difficult conversations and ultimately, the catalyst that brings us fully into our light and the best versions of ourselves.

Rozanne, Rochelle's Niece

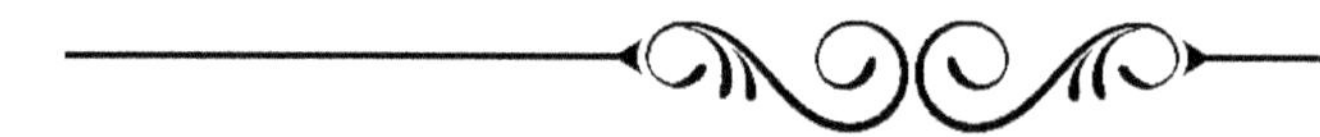

A journey of love, integrity and finding your true self.

Rochelle bears all in this story of love, letting go, and profound spiritual healing. Growing up in South Africa during apartheid, attempting to navigate complex societal expectations from a young age, her journey is one of vulnerability and courage, lighting the way and inviting the reader to follow her on their search to discover their true selves. Rochelle's story is uplifting, a jarring yet liberating reminder that life is about choices, and no matter what conditions are forced upon us, we can find peace when we live in alignment with our authentic values and beliefs. I am privileged to know Rochelle personally, first as my boss, mentor, and now as family. When I first met her in a corporate setting, she stood out. She was never afraid to challenge the status quo. Her integrity and moral compass defined her actions and always kept her true to herself. The corporate world can be savage, and Rochelle is too good for It. As I once wrote in an employee survey, *"Integrity walked out the door with Rochelle Trow."* Rochelle deeply believes that "we rise by lifting others," and she has lifted me, changing my life as I have seen her do with so many people. This story is about her own self-discovery, but to me, she is finally recognising the remarkable person I've seen and admired all along.

Emily Murphy, friend who has become family

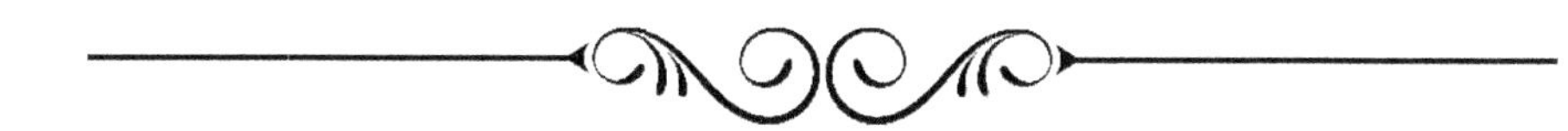

When dancing in the rain becomes the pathway to freedom

I have known Rochelle in both a professional and a personal capacity for close to twenty years. In that time, what has consistently shone through is her drive, her tenacity, her openness and sheer courage.

When Rochelle took part in a project during lockdown called the Butterfly Effect, we talked about a shift from an all-consuming drive to achieve to instead being guided by an inner sense of being. In true Rochelle style, when realisation later dawned that she was not living her life with true authenticity, she chose to confront what was standing in the way of that reality and her future happiness. It meant consciously and courageously stripping back the numerous layers of protection that she had put in place over the years and embracing the person she found within. Five years later, the answer is clear. Rochelle has made the transition. She truly has learnt to dance in the rain. She is now in touch with her sense of self. She knows her true self-worth and fully embraces what life brings her with joy in her heart. Moreover, she is clear on what she can do to help those others who have also reached that point of no return in their life's journey. Awakening to Wholeness: a Life Unmasked is a must-read. It is a call to action for those business leaders, professionals, parents and all those caught in a maelstrom and struggling to live their full and authentic lives. It showcases Rochelle's extraordinary journey and what is ultimately possible for those who dare while simultaneously inviting readers to embrace their own path to freedom. As Rochelle demonstrates, it is a journey that is worth fighting for.

Christine D'Mello, coach, chef, writer and friend who has become family

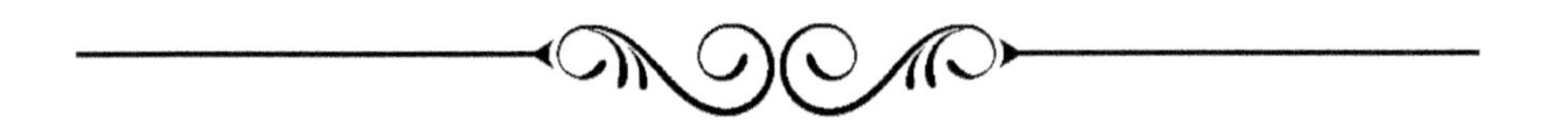

Awakening to Wholeness: A Journey That Feels Like Coming Home

For over 22 years, Rochelle and I have weathered storms, lifted each other high, dried tears, laughed until our sides ached, and loved each other deeply—not just as friends but as family.

Rochelle's journey—her relentless drive to become the best version of herself spiritually, mentally, and physically—is truly inspiring. Her book speaks authentically to the heart, offering hope, practical insights, and gentle encouragement for personal growth.

As someone who has leaned on Rochelle's empathy and wisdom during my own challenges, I can attest to her ability to guide and uplift. Her reflections on love, resilience, and the complexities of relationships resonated deeply with me, echoing my own experiences of navigating self-doubt and healing.

This book is not prescriptive but empowering. Rochelle shines a light on the path to healing, inviting readers to reflect, shift mindsets, and embrace their true selves. Even if you've never met her, her sincerity and warmth will leap off the page, inspiring you to explore your journey.

Rochelle, thank you for being my anchor and a beacon in every storm. Your book is a gift, and I am proud to call you my sister.

Emma Sinclair Family in every way that matters

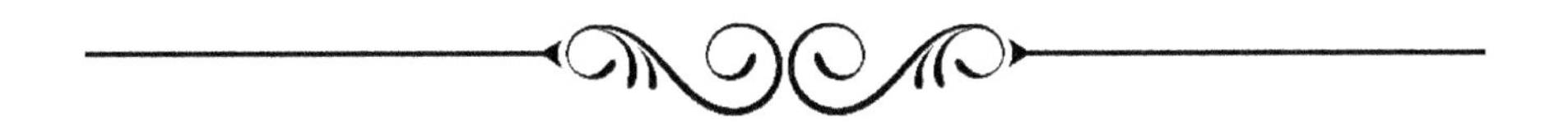

Food for the Soul.

This book takes us on an intimate pilgrimage along the road less travelled, peeling away the layers to uncover our true selves in the process.

I've had the privilege of knowing Rochelle for 23 years. Our paths first crossed as fellow South Africans and colleagues across two very different industries, and in time, we forged a deeply cherished friendship.

Much like a butterfly symbolises transformation, rebirth, and growth, this book embodies Rochelle's journey of self-discovery and her courage to change, evolve, and inspire.

For anyone embarking on their own path of self-discovery, this is an essential read. Each chapter invites reflection and offers profound insights that are both relatable and uplifting. Rochelle's raw honesty and authenticity make this book not only inspiring but also nourishing for the soul.

I couldn't wait to turn each page and uncover the next chapter of her extraordinary story.

Janine Canterbury Director, Coach & Autoimmune Patient Advocate

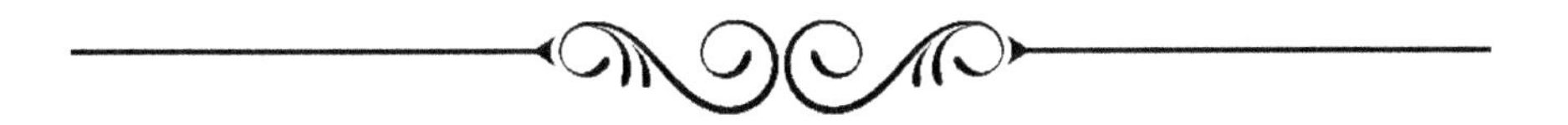

TABLE OF CONTENTS

INTRODUCTION

Invitation to the Reader

Every journey is unique, and while this isn't a self-help book, I hope that by sharing my story, you might find something that stirs your own reflections. When I sit quietly, I often feel immense gratitude, grounded by the deep love I have for my twin boys. They are the bright lights guiding me out of the shadows where I once felt lost, helping me reconnect with myself. This book is a heartfelt monument of joy, sorrow, struggle, and triumph — a collection of moments that capture my journey.

Why Tell This Story?

This story explores the delicate line between the roles we take on in life and the essence of who we truly are. For years, I moulded myself to fit what society expected, letting the world shape my identity while ignoring the vibrant spirit within me. My career blossomed, and we enjoyed financial comfort, but despite the success, my happiness faded. I felt like a ghost, trapped in a life that no longer fit.

Through this book, I want to share the intricacies of my quest — not only to rediscover my true self but to turn past pain into a source of light and authenticity. This story is a testament to the strength of the human spirit and the life-changing power of self-love. It honours the courageous journey of accepting who we truly are, marked by vulnerability and the firm belief that each of us deserves love and joy.

A Reflection of My Life

As you read these pages, you'll step into my world — a reflection of my life as I've experienced it. We each see life through our unique lens, shaped by our individual experiences and emotions. While others may remember certain moments differently, this is my story, and I want to share my journey, with all its layers and shades.

Drawing on my love for poetry, I begin each chapter with a poem that captures the heart of the chapter. These poems are crafted from my own words and enhanced with generative AI to give each one the essence of what I want to convey.

In telling this story, I've tried to balance openness and respect for privacy. When someone has asked for anonymity, I've honoured their wishes by changing names and softening details. But for the family and friends who have given me permission to share our experiences as they are, their names remain — a reminder of the connections we've built.

The heart of this book is centred on my life after 2019, though I sometimes revisit earlier years that deeply shaped my transformation. This story weaves together moments of uncertainty and clarity, strengthened by challenges that shaped my identity — from the shadows of self-doubt to the bright light of self-discovery. Here, I recount the struggles that redefined my life, including the quiet victories that helped me reclaim my voice.

A Journey of Reflection

The tone of this book is reflective, inviting you to walk with me as I navigate a profound transformation. I encourage you to consider your own journey toward authenticity, finding your voice amidst the noise of others' expectations. This story is not just a record of events; it's an invitation to connect with the raw, unfiltered reality of the human experience.

As we go deeper, I hope you find yourself in moments of clarity, struggle, and growth that echo our shared desire to live genuinely. Let's embark on this journey of understanding, healing, and self-discovery together, honouring the beauty and complexity within our lives. Let my story be a reminder for anyone who's ever felt lost — a reminder that the power to reclaim who we truly are lies within us all.

In the following poem, I hope to capture the spirit of this book — a guiding anthem for anyone who's ever felt adrift, showing that we all have the strength to rediscover our true selves. As you turn the pages, I invite you to walk beside me on this path of transformation, finding the beauty and strength that come from embracing your own light.

In a world where expectations weigh heavy,

I walked through life sturdy and steady,

A woman shaped by society's mould,

My true self hidden, my story left untold.

With twin boys and a husband so vain,

Financial freedom yet burdened with pain,

I lost myself in roles I played,

My spirit dulled, my heart dismayed.

Day after day, I played the part,

But deep inside, I felt torn apart,

My soul yearned to break free and fly,

To answer the question: Who am I?

In the mirror, a stranger stared back,

Lost in the shadows, off the beaten track,

My true essence buried deep within,

Awaiting rediscovery to let my journey begin.

Through trials and tears, I found my way,

Unveiling the mask, embracing the day,

I let go of expectations, embraced my truth,

Reconnecting with myself, the essence of my youth.

With newfound courage, I learned to be,

Authentic, bold, and finally free,

No longer defined by others' views,

But by the light within, my spirit infused.

So, let my story be a guiding anthem,

For all who've forgotten to truly fathom,

The power within to shine bright and high,

And reclaim the answer to the question: Who am I

Prologue: Life and a Dance of Roles

In the tapestry of life, I wear many threads,

A wife with tender love, where my heart gently spreads,

Balancing warmth with the weight of the day,

In quiet moments, I seek to find my way.

As a mother, I nurture, my heart in each hand,

Guiding little lives, like grains of soft sand,

With laughter and lessons, I build their bright dreams,

Yet, in their joy, I sometimes lose my own gleams.

As a sister, I cherish the bonds we have spun,

In shared laughter and tears, our lives intertwine as one,

Yet, in the shadows, I wrestle with guilt,

For the time that slips by, like a house that I built.

As an aunt, I'm a beacon, a source of delight,

With stories and hugs that make everything right,

But beneath the smiles, a longing resides,

To give all my love, while my own self hides.

In the boardroom, I stand, an executive bold,

Where strategies flourish, and ambitions unfold,

Yet behind the sharp suit, I carry the strain,

Of juggling these roles, a delicate chain.

Each title I wear pulls me in different ways,

Insecurity whispers, filling my days,

"Am I doing enough? Will they see my flaws?"

In the depths of my mind, self-doubt fiercely claws.

The fear of not being good enough looms,

As I chase the bright dreams amidst unseen glooms,

I strive for success, yet it feels like a race,

A constant reminder of the roles I embrace.

In the quiet of night, when the world fades away,

I gather my fragments, piece by piece, day by day,

For in this complex weave, I seek to be whole,

A tapestry rich with the hues of my soul.

Yet, the struggle remains, a dance of despair,

To balance my worth with the love that I bear,

In this whirlwind of life, with its joy and its pain,

I learn to find strength in the heart of the strain.

When I sat down to write this book, memories came flooding back, reminding me of the delicate line between the roles I've played and who I truly am deep down. For so long, I conformed to the relentless demands of societal expectations, letting the world shape me while ignoring the lively, real self that I kept buried. My career was successful, and we enjoyed financial freedom, yet beneath it all, my happiness faded. I felt like a ghost of my true self, trapped in a role that no longer felt right.

The pages ahead serve as a short introduction to the deeper journey that follows. Each chapter will explore moments that shaped who I am and transformed my spirit. Step by step, I'll pull back the layers of my story, sharing the struggles and victories that have defined me in ways I never imagined.

For years, I felt like an outsider — a shadow at the edge of every room. It was easier to say what others wanted to hear than to show my true thoughts and feelings. Little did I know how this choice would shape my life, leading me to a place of frustration and emptiness. Over time, I grew to dislike the person I saw in the mirror — someone who had lost her inner voice. This inner struggle affected my relationships, even with my own children, echoing back to me in ways that left my heart aching.

My story starts in South Africa, where I was the youngest in a large family of eleven siblings. Growing up in such a busy household, I often felt invisible among the noise of laughter, arguments, and everyday life. With so many voices around me, I craved attention but rarely received it — except when my frustration boiled over and led to emotional outbursts. When I did manage to grab a bit of my family's attention, I often felt misunderstood, like a piece of the puzzle that didn't quite fit. I learned to hold back my real feelings, showing only what I thought would make others happy. This became my way of protecting myself from the pain of being overlooked.

In my family, love was shown through actions and spending time together, but to me, it often felt heavy and a bit forced, lacking the warmth I longed for. I began to wonder if we were really connecting or just competing for each other's affection. Even in "quality time," I felt like we were each fighting to be heard. While my siblings voiced their opinions, I withdrew, finding it easier to be quiet and watch from the sidelines — feeling both safer and lonelier at the same time, a quiet observer in a world that seemed to move on without me.

My sense of not fitting in extended into my community. While other teens were caught up in gossip and dating, I felt different — I just wanted to be myself, even if I wasn't sure who that was. Trying to fit in with the local coloured community, all of us bearing the weight of apartheid, I went through years of chemical treatments to straighten my hair. I tried hard to conform to a beauty ideal that felt both distant and uncomfortable. Every treatment, with its sharp smell of chemicals, was a reminder of my desire to belong. But even after all that, I never felt like it filled the emptiness inside. I'd look in the mirror and see someone who didn't quite look like me — a stranger wearing a mask that didn't feel right.

The church, too, became a point of struggle in my life. Growing up in a religious home full of rituals and traditions, I started to feel disconnected from these practices as I got older. I wanted a direct, personal relationship with God, one that didn't need rituals or intermediaries. In my heart, I felt alone in these beliefs, afraid to speak out because I didn't want to be rejected. The church, which should have been a place of comfort, became yet another place where I hid my true self, buried under layers of others' expectations.

School felt like another battleground where I struggled with my sense of identity. I remember sitting in classrooms focused on memorising facts and repeating them — this style bored me and left me craving something more. I wanted real, hands-on experiences that encouraged me to think deeply and discover myself. But instead of finding inspiration, I often felt like I didn't belong, drifting in a sea of disinterest. When I got to university, I was one of the few non-white students at a campus still carrying remnants of apartheid. My impoverished high school education didn't prepare me well for a university once open only to white students. The pressure to fit in felt overwhelming, and I developed a crippling sense of inferiority. Rather than speaking up, I stayed silent, afraid to ask questions for fear of looking stupid or showing how lost I sometimes felt. Walking through the campus, I tried to blend in, feeling like a ghost among others who seemed so at ease — just wishing to be seen, to be heard, to take my place in the world.

When I moved to London and later Switzerland, I hoped for fresh starts but only felt more lost. Michael Singer's words in *The Untethered Soul* struck a chord with me: "You are not your thoughts; you are the one who observes your thoughts." This made me realise that the front I put on was just that — a carefully crafted image to meet the expectations of others. Outwardly, I seemed confident and composed, like I wore a mask of bravery. But inside, my mind was full of doubts that clashed with my actions. The more I forced myself to conform to society's expectations, the further I drifted from my true self. Singer's advice helped me step back and observe my thoughts without judgment, guiding me toward a more authentic way of living.

In the corporate world, I often found myself as one of the few women — or sometimes the only one — on executive leadership teams dominated by men. The weight of the stereotypes I'd grown to resent pressed down on me. Although I was raised to stand up to injustice, I often silenced myself to avoid disrupting the established order. Ironically, even in my Human Resources team, where women were the majority, I sometimes faced the same behaviours I thought only men displayed, with some women exhibiting more combative tendencies than I'd expected.

During those early years in my career, diversity seemed like an idea that was out of reach. I remember feeling frustrated by the injustices I saw but often pulled back from conflicts instead of facing them head-on. My lack of confidence became a crutch, allowing me to stay in the background while the harsh realities of corporate life shaped my decisions. Rather than use my voice to fight for change, I convinced myself it was safer to stay quiet. Even now, while discussions about diversity have evolved, I sometimes feel torn about the agenda, especially when it seems that some people hold onto a victim mindset instead of empowering themselves. Many of us have faced racism and stereotyping but have risen above it.

At work dinners, as colleagues talked about fancy vacations and lavish lifestyles, I felt my own life shrink in comparison. Every story around the table highlighted my own insecurities and made me feel small. I stayed silent, just listening as they bonded, afraid that sharing my own stories would lead to judgment or, worse, pity. So, I nodded along, all the while feeling a mixture of envy and shame in my heart.

One of my biggest secrets was that I couldn't swim — a fear stemming from a childhood experience that left me paralysed with anxiety. Just the thought of social events involving water, like beach trips or pool parties, felt like facing a wall I couldn't climb. I avoided those gatherings entirely, never wanting to admit my fear, which only deepened my sense of isolation.

As a mother, the pressure to fit in only grew stronger. School pickups, parent-teacher meetings, and casual chats with other parents at my kids' private school became a source of anxiety. The worry of being judged or standing out because of my perceived flaws made me nervous. I craved connection with others but felt trapped by my insecurities, too afraid to reach out.

Moving to Switzerland felt like stepping into a beautiful, fresh chapter of my life. The heavy weight I'd carried for so long started to lift. Surrounded by breathtaking landscapes, serene lakes, and the towering Alps, I felt as though I was being given a fresh start — a blank canvas where I could create the life I truly wanted.

For years, I felt like life's challenges controlled me, and I built walls around my heart to protect myself from disappointment. As Michael Singer points out in *The Untethered Soul*, we often close ourselves off, going into a defensive mode that keeps us from experiencing the fullness of life. But in the calm of Switzerland, I began to see things differently. The beauty around me gave me the clarity I needed. In that peaceful corner of the world, I began to question everything — my choices, my relationships, and, most importantly, myself. With each moment of reflection, I felt those walls start to crumble, letting the light of understanding seep in.

The journey of self-discovery wasn't easy. Pulling back the layers of protection I'd built felt overwhelming at first. I'd grown used to the safety of my cocoon, even if it was stifling. But as I settled into my new surroundings, a deep longing emerged — a desire to reconnect with the person I had hidden away under all that self-protection. Tara Brach expresses it perfectly when she says, "The most fundamental healing we can do is to reconnect with our true self, to feel the love and compassion that is our essence." The beauty of the Swiss landscape mirrored the potential I saw in myself. Slowly, I began to unravel my past, facing the fears that had kept me from truly living.

One of the hardest truths I had to face was the reality of my marriage. For twenty years, I held on to the hope that love could be the glue to keep us together. But when I started my new life, I could finally see the unhealthy patterns in my marriage more clearly. The narcissistic behaviour I had been trying to overlook was suddenly undeniable. It was a harsh wake-up call that, though it came late, I needed to see. My husband and I weren't helping each other grow; we were trapped in a cycle of hurt and emotional distance. The idea of leaving scared me, but staying felt even harder. As I dealt with these realisations, I also started to look at my other relationships more closely. The wound I carried from childhood left emotional scars that influenced how I connected with others. I began to notice how certain relationships stirred up old wounds, pulling me back into toxic dynamics. This was painful to realise, but I knew it was necessary to acknowledge. Dr. Perry and Oprah Winfrey say it well: "The experiences we have in our early years shape our capacity for empathy, connection, and resilience." Learning to let go of these harmful relationships — especially in a workplace full of self-centred people — became a key part of my healing. I had to choose my own well-being over the fear of judgment or loss.

Through this self-reflection, I discovered something powerful: I didn't need to fit in; I needed to be real. I had spent too long trying to become what I thought others expected of me. But in Switzerland, I finally felt free to be myself. I learned that I didn't need anyone's approval to be worthy. I didn't have to be loud to be seen or pretend to be something I wasn't. This was liberating and helped me let go of insecurities I had carried for years.

As I began to take charge of my thoughts and feelings, I felt a new confidence growing. I realised it was okay to ask for help, to reach out for support, and to be kind to myself. Tara Brach's words from "Radical Compassion" hit home for me: "Compassion is the radicalism of our time." Each small act of kindness toward myself felt like a victory — a sign that I was moving forward. I started investing in my personal growth, taking on challenges that pushed me out of my comfort zone. I sought therapy, practised mindfulness, and surrounded myself with people who lifted me up. Every step I took reminded me of my strength and my ability to change.

Switzerland became my safe haven — a place where I could truly breathe and think. In that calm, I learned to listen to my own heart again. I found that real peace comes from living in alignment with who you are, not from meeting others' expectations. I learned that it's okay to walk away from things that don't bring you joy, even if it feels hard. I realised I had the power to create my own happiness, without needing approval from others.

As I continue on this journey, I hold on to the insights I've gained. I now understand that there's strength in being vulnerable, value in standing up for myself, and freedom in letting go of things that hold me back. I'm no longer wandering lost; I'm uncovering who I've always been, one step at a time. Each day in Switzerland brings a new chance to live my truth, celebrate my growth, and honour the experiences that have shaped me.

In the beauty of these mountains and lakes, I'm learning to love myself deeply. I understand that it's okay to fall down as long as I keep getting up, a little stronger each time. As poet Rupi Kaur says, "How you love yourself is how you teach others to love you." Looking back, I see a pattern in my life — a deep need to belong and be accepted, often at the cost of being true to myself. The journey to authenticity has been long and painful, and it's still ongoing.

This experience of feeling like an outsider has changed me in ways I'm only beginning to grasp. It's left marks of pain and longing, but it's also sparked a strong desire to find my true self. As I reflect on all of this, I see these memories as more than just chapters from my past; they are stepping stones to a more genuine life. Every struggle, every time I felt left out, has shaped who I am today. It's pushed me to rise up, reclaim my voice, and embrace the beauty of my journey — imperfections and all.

How Lineage and Society Shape Our Identity

Moving Forward with Gratitude: Honouring Our Roots

Ode to Generations Past

In the soft whispers of the evening breeze,

I sense the presence of those who came before,

Three generations intertwined in life's design,

Their threads of bravery and strength evermore.

From hands that worked under the sun's warm glow,

To hearts that nurtured dreams with gentle care,

Each tale inscribed upon the fabric's weave,

In love's embrace, their spirits linger there.

Thank you, cherished ancestors, for your guiding light,

For teaching me to stand, to rise, to strive,

Through every trial, your wisdom stood so tall,

In each challenge faced, I hear your call.

Your laughter swirls in the autumn leaves,

Your tears have nourished the roots of my soul,

With every lesson, my heart believes,

That love and joy together make us whole.

You passed down values like a sacred flame,

In kindness and resilience, you paved the way,

With open hearts, you embraced life's joy and pain,

In your warmth, I find strength each day.

So, here's my gratitude, a simple song,

For the legacy of love that you shared,

In every step I take, I carry along,

The essence of your spirit, always prepared.

May I honour you in all that I pursue,

With courage, strength, and joy as my guide,

For in my heart, I hold each of you,

Three generations strong, forever by my side.

As I take a moment to think about my life, I'm filled with a deep sense of gratitude. I can't put in words how much I owe to the generations before me. My life feels like part of a larger story, each of us connected by the lives of those who came before. Each person has added something to who I am, and I don't want to overlook the remarkable lineage that has shaped me. Let me take you on a journey through my family's history. My father's side has a long and well-documented past that goes way back. I'm especially grateful to my aunt, Viva Lewey, for her incredible book, *Thunder from a Clear Sky*. Her writing opened up a window into this rich history, and it inspired me to dig deeper and share the story of my father's family.

On my mother's side, the story isn't as clearly outlined, but it's just as lively. Through stories passed down from my aunts and uncles to my older siblings, I've been able to piece together a beautiful mosaic of our past. I'm especially thankful to my sister Merle for her dedication to tracing our family tree. Thanks to her, I've been able to gather moments and memories that really speak to me. The stories of the Trow and Butka families echo within me, showing just how connected I am to their legacies.

Writing this chapter has taught me something important: so much of who I am today reflects the lives of those who came before me. It's humbling to realise this. I have to admit, when I was younger, I didn't fully understand just how much my parents shaped who I am. But as I write my book, I'm seeing things from a new perspective. I've been able to revisit the beloved stories my siblings shared with me, and through them, I see pieces of my mom and dad within me—more than I ever noticed as a child.

Though it pains me that they are no longer with us, I am determined to honour their memory. This chapter is not just a tribute to my parents but to all the generations who came before me. Their sacrifices, struggles, and triumphs built the foundation of my life. I may not have the chance to tell them how much they mean to me, but through these words, I hope to show them the depth of my love and gratitude.

By celebrating our past, I'm embracing the truth that we are deeply shaped by those who came before us. Their stories live on in us, lighting the way forward. As I piece together my family's history, I do it with a heart full of gratitude—thankful for every voice that has echoed through the years, reminding me of where I come from and who I am destined to be.

MY FAMILY TREE

GREAT-GREAT GRANDPARENTS
SAMUEL MACKIN PEDLAR
ELLEN COX
CHILDREN

GREAT-GREAT GRANDPARENTS
GEORGE TROW
UNNAMED WIFE
CHILDREN

GREAT GRANDPARENTS
SOPHIA KATE PEDLAR
ELLEN MARY
ALICE
GEORGE JUNIOR
JAMES THOMAS TROW

GRANDPARENTS
HARRY (GRAND FATHER) 4th BORN
JOSEPHINE (GRAND MOTHER)
9 OTHERS SIBLINGS
CHILDREN
SPALDING JOSEPH TROW (DAD)
JOYCE
ALBERT

GRANDPARENTS
AMOD EBRAHIM BUTKA (PENNY)
JANET GABAGAS
CHILDREN
LILY ROSALIE BUTKA (MOM)
EVA
EBRAHIM (JOHNNY)

PARENTS

EUGENE

JENNIFER
CHILDREN
ZEIDAH
IGSAAN

MARLYN
CHILDREN
DALENE
NATALIE

MERLE
CHILDREN
MARC
CARRYN
ALAIN

DAWN
CHILDREN
MELANIE
DEON
ROBBYN

ALVIN
CHILDREN
MELVIN
RICARDO

KEITH
CHILDREN
ROZANNE
ARLENE

CLAUDETTE
CHILDREN
DANE
CODY
ARNE

SHERWIN
CHILDREN
TORI LEIGH
TYRA DANAE

LAVERN
CHILDREN
SHERAZAAD
ASHLEY

ROCHELLE (MARRIED EMMETT IN 2001)
CHILDREN
TYSON
ZACH

Lineage and Family History of the Trows

As I look back on my family's history, a rich bundle of stories unfolds before me, filled with resilience, love, and the unbreakable spirit of my ancestors. This story begins with George Trow, my great-great-grandfather, who left his home in England in the mid-1800s. I picture him—a determined man with big dreams—making the long journey to South Africa with his wife and four children, two boys, and two girls, holding onto hope in the face of the unknown.

They made their new home in East London, where George first tried his hand at farming. But he found his true calling when he established the Trows Inn in Umtata. I imagine the inn, full of life and laughter, becoming a place where my family's roots began to grow. However, tragedy struck when George and his wife both passed away early on, leaving their sons, James and George Junior, to face a tough world on their own. Forced to grow up quickly, they sold newspapers and went to night school, driven by a thirst for knowledge and a need to survive.

Then there was Ellen Cox, my great-great-grandmother, who started her journey in Cobh, County Cork, Ireland. Born during the devastating potato famine, Ellen represented the courage of many Irish people looking for a better life. She left everything she knew, working as a governess in England, where her education opened doors for her. When the opportunity came for young women to go to South Africa to marry British soldiers, Ellen didn't hesitate. I can almost hear her laughter on that first meeting with Samuel Peglar, the soldier she would marry. They had three daughters together, including Sophia Kate, my great-grandmother.

Sophia Kate, born in 1858, carried her family's legacy with her when she married James Trow, my great-grandfather. Their love grew during the struggles of the 1870s, and they had ten children together. I often think of the energy and joy that must have filled their home in Collywobbles, near Butterworth. But life wasn't easy; they eventually had to flee Engcobo due to tribal conflicts. Losing their home and livelihood must have felt overwhelming, but James stayed resilient, working at his brother's trading station to support his family.

James was more than just strong—he was a respected figure in his community. I can see him, standing proud even at the age of 84, with his love for sailing and his time served in the military during the Xhosa and Zulu wars showing his sense of purpose and courage.

Sophie Kate, my great-grandmother, was the heart of their bustling household. I imagine her surrounded by the noise and laughter of her ten children, always busy with cooking, baking, and caring for everyone. She filled their lives with homemade jams, canned fruits, and a sense of abundance. The land they worked together flourished, filled with oranges, lemons, and a variety of other fruits, while the animals they raised became part of their family's story.

Yet life also brought its lows. In 1918, Sophie Kate passed away from breast cancer at the age of 60, leaving behind a legacy of love that still lives within me. I often find myself reflecting on the sacrifices and resilience of these remarkable ancestors who laid the groundwork for my own life. Their journey through hardship and heartache, love and laughter, stands as a powerful reminder of family strength.

As I continue to piece together my family's story, my heart swells with both pride and sadness, especially when I think of the story of Harry and Josephine. My grandfather, Harry Trow, was born in 1882 in the small village of Engcobo in the Transkei. He was the fourth son of James and Kate Trow, a lively spirit in a large family of ten. His childhood was full of the vibrant colours of the land—lush, green, and alive with the spirit of the Xhosa people.

Growing up in the Transkei wasn't easy. Harry and his siblings moved from village to village, uprooted by the clan conflicts that sometimes flared among the Xhosa. But amidst these difficult times, they found comfort in the beauty around them. Eventually, they settled in Thembuland when their father bought Qingqolo in 1903, a piece of land that would become central to their lives. Here, at the Orange

Grove homestead, they learned to live off the land—growing fruit and vegetables and taking care of cattle, pigs, sheep, and chickens.

Harry's childhood was filled with adventure. He and his siblings, White children in an African land, formed friendships with the local Xhosa kids. They swam in rivers, their laughter echoing off the water, and raced on horseback across the fields. I can almost see them, carefree under the sun, racing towards the horizon. Their holidays in Coffee Bay and Port St. Johns were filled with the salty ocean air and the warmth of family gatherings.

Education, however, was a challenge. The nearest school was 13 kilometres away, and sometimes they had to cross a river that, when swollen with rain, made the village unreachable. Despite these obstacles, Harry's younger siblings were taught at home by their older sister, who had trained as a governess. I wonder how Harry felt about his education, especially compared to his brother Gordon, who went on to become a well-known lawyer in Umtata. Harry, on the other hand, found his path as a tradesman, working in his father's store.

In my search through Harry's life, I come across hints of his time in the military, but it's his colourful escapades that capture my imagination. He would disappear for weeks, wrapped in a blanket, joining the tribal red blanket people for camaraderie and drinks. It was during one of these gatherings that he met my grandmother, Josephine, a strong Xhosa woman from the Red Blanket People. Their love, although socially frowned upon, blossomed quietly in a world that wasn't ready for them.

Josephine was a remarkable woman. My dad remembers her as a mix of tradition and change—she had converted to Christianity and wore full skirts in deep blue and white, reflecting her gentle spirit. As an unmarried mother, she raised their three children, Albert, Joyce, and Spalding, in four interconnected rondavels on a small hill in Ndulini, just a few kilometres from the Trow homestead. Harry visited regularly, making sure they had food, warmth, and an education, even when society ignored their family.

Tragedy struck in 1936 when Harry died at only 54. The cause of his death remains a mystery, with rumours of him drowning in a river or dying in a car accident. Josephine and their eldest son, Albert, also died with him, leaving Joyce and Spalding orphaned. It breaks my heart to think of their loss—two parents gone too soon, their love story fading into whispers.

The silence that surrounded Harry's relationship with Josephine, his family's rejection, and the harshness of apartheid in South Africa weigh heavily on me. In a time when mixed-race relationships were scorned, their love stood as a quiet act of defiance. It saddens me to think that James and Kate Trow likely disowned their son and his family, unable to accept the unique legacy that Harry and Josephine created together.

But as I recount these stories, I feel a deep connection to my roots. Harry and Josephine's love story, despite its hardships, speaks to my own identity. Their legacy lives on in me—a reminder of the strength that love can bring against prejudice and tradition. By sharing their story, I honour not only their memory but the essence of who I am.

As I trace my family's lines, I am filled with gratitude for the resilience that runs through my veins. Their stories aren't just history; they are the essence of who I am. In honouring my heritage, I find a deep sense of love, connection, and pride that drives me forward, reminding me that I am a part of this beautiful picture painted by the Trows and Peglars.

Spalding Joseph Trow (My Dad)

I remember my father, Spalding, as a strong, resilient man whose life was woven with hard work and love. He was born on March 19, 1923, in Thembuland, Transkei, as the child of a mixed-race relationship. His father, Harry, was white, and his mother, Josephine, was Xhosa. Dad grew up in traditional round huts on a small hill in Ndulini, living with his mother and siblings while his father visited regularly to support them and bridge the gap between their two worlds.

Dad started school at a local African primary school in Nqwara, and later moved to another school in Qokolweni. Grandpa Harry didn't agree with this decision, wanting the best opportunities for his children. So he enrolled Dad as a boarder at the Holy Cross Convent School at Circira, just outside Umtata. But when Dad was only 13, tragedy struck — he lost his father, brother, and mother in quick succession in 1936. Left to face the world on his own, he stayed at the convent until he was sixteen.

In 1939, with World War II beginning, Dad joined the army, volunteering for the Cape Coloured Corps. His service took him from Cape Town to North Africa, where he joined the Signal Corps. His duties included building bridges and roads for advancing troops. He travelled through Ethiopia, Sudan, Cairo, Libya, and even served with a French regiment in France before moving on to Britain. These experiences deeply shaped him, giving him resilience and skills that would later serve him well in civilian life.

After the war, Dad returned to Umtata, where he used his skills in construction. A wealthy lawyer hired him to manage building projects at trading stations across the area. With determination, he saved enough money to move to Durban and start his own construction company, "Trow Construction." This marked a new chapter in his life, both professionally and personally.

Dad met my mother, Lily Rosalie Butka, during a weekend trip to Matatiele with a friend from the military. Their connection grew quickly, and they married in 1949. Together, they began a journey that would bring them eleven children. In their early years in Durban, they lived in a modest outbuilding, where they welcomed their first children, including my siblings Jennifer, Marlyn, and Merle. Sadly, their firstborn, Eugene, passed away as an infant.

In 1954, Dad bought land in Sparks Estate with a dream to build a home for our growing family. He spent every spare moment working on our house at 14 Mary Road, often staying up late and working on weekends. By 1956, we moved into our new home, and soon after, my sister Dawn was born. Our family became mostly self-sufficient, growing our own vegetables, fruit, and eggs from our chickens, thanks to Dad's resourcefulness.

As a building contractor, Dad's work often took him far from home to places like Zululand, Pinetown, and Pietermaritzburg. Despite being away so much, he was well-known in the community for his honesty and kindness. Although he wasn't the shrewdest businessman, he was generous to a fault, sometimes missing payments from clients who took advantage of his kindness. Dad valued education deeply, insisting on quality schooling for all of us, even enrolling the oldest at a respected boarding school in Ixopo.

Our family grew with the arrivals of Elvin, Keith, Claudette, Sherwin, Lavern, and finally me, Rochelle. Dad was adventurous and sometimes would disappear for long stretches, much to Mom's frustration. Twice he was even declared dead, only to reappear later. These disappearances, while worrying, became part of his larger-than-life character, echoing stories we'd heard about Grandpa Harry.

In the mid-1990s, a surprising encounter brought us in touch with Dad's white relatives. I met my second cousin Sandy at a Woolworths food market, reconnecting us with Dad's white family. This reunion was bittersweet, as it took almost a lifetime for Dad to be accepted by his white relatives. But he harboured no resentment, embracing the new South Africa with grace. With the end of apartheid, our family was finally recognised as rightful descendants of the James Trow family.

Even in his later years, Dad continued working on construction sites, climbing scaffolds well into his seventies. He was unwaveringly determined, and every moment with family was precious to him. But as he aged, his eyesight began to fail, and without a driver's license, he had to slow down, which was a hard adjustment for him, as he struggled with the loss of independence.

In 2005, our family was shaken when Dad was diagnosed with prostate cancer. We were heartbroken, especially knowing it had already spread to his liver. Yet Dad made a brave choice: he declined medical treatment, choosing instead to rely on palliative care. He faced his illness with incredible strength, refusing painkillers or sedatives. It seemed he wanted to experience every moment, no matter how painful, on his own terms. His resilience inspired us, though it was painful to see him endure this battle alone.

As months passed, we gathered around him, sharing stories and memories, trying to fill each day with love and laughter. But we all felt the weight of what was coming. Six months after his diagnosis, on February 21, 2006, we said our final goodbye to Spalding, just four weeks before his 84th birthday. His passing left a void in our hearts and reminded us of the strength and courage of a man who faced life, and his final moments, with unmatched grace.

The Butka Family Lineage and History

Thinking about the Butka family history fills me with pride and admiration. My grandfather, Amod Ebrahim Butka — known fondly as Penny — had a story of courage, determination, and hard work that shaped our family's journey.

Our story begins in Gujarat, India, a place rich with tradition and culture. At just 12 years old, Penny took a big step that would change his life forever. Out of necessity and a sense of adventure, he hid on a ship carrying workers to the sugar plantations of Natal, South Africa. This journey, filled with challenges and unknowns, was the start of his incredible life.

When he was discovered on the ship, Penny was put to work cleaning and sweeping. He earned his nickname by diligently picking up every penny he found. Even at that young age, his resourcefulness and hard work were clear—qualities that would define his future.

As fate would have it, the ship wrecked in Cape Town, saving Penny from the hard life of plantation work. Now stranded in a new land, he met Mr. Goga, a fellow traveller, who offered him support. Living with the Goga family in District Six, Penny learned important entrepreneurial skills that would help him later in life.

Penny eventually made his way to Kokstad, where he met my grandmother, Janet Gabagas. Their meeting was by chance, but it led to a lifelong partnership. Janet and Penny married young and moved to Matatiele, a town with a rugged charm near Matatiele Mountain.

Here, Penny's entrepreneurial spirit truly flourished. Using the skills he'd learned, he built a successful hardware store and later, a legal firm. His businesses thrived, a testament to his sharp mind and hard work. With his earnings, he bought a piece of land on Station Road, creating a home that became a family sanctuary. The property included two houses, orchards filled with fruit trees, and wide gardens—a symbol of his hard work and vision.

Though there's less known about my grandmother Janet's life, her role was equally important. Born in Kokstad as one of six children, she shared a background of resilience and strength. She met Penny when she was young, and together, they built a life filled with love and purpose. Janet dedicated herself to raising their three children — Ebrahim, Eva, and my mother, Lily Rosalie — with strong values in faith, family, and community.

Janet's days were busy with the routines of family life. She took care of her garden, cooked hearty meals, and cared for her children. Her garden's roses and the warmth of her kitchen are cherished memories for those who knew her. Janet's strength held the family together, especially after Penny's sudden death in his mid-forties. She became the glue that bound the family, her spirit unwavering.

Through Penny and Janet's story, I see the values of perseverance and resilience. Their legacy isn't just about surviving hard times; it's about thriving and creating a future for the family. They built a foundation for the Butka family that allows future generations to grow and succeed.

Looking back on their journey fills me with gratitude and inspiration. Their sacrifices and accomplishments are part of our family's history, shaping who we are. As I carry on their legacy, I am reminded of the strength of resilience, love, and the human spirit. Their story is a source of hope and strength for us all.

Lily Rosalie Trow (née Butka) – My Mother

As I reflect on my life, I am surrounded by memories of my mother, Lily. Born in the quiet town of Matatiele on April 10th 1930, she was the youngest of three siblings. Her childhood was full of family, faith, and joy. I picture her as a spirited little girl, surrounded by fruit trees and laughter, with the love of her parents, Penny and Janet.

Growing up on a smallholding, Lily's childhood was filled with the smells of ripening peaches, plums, and apricots. I imagine her as a carefree child, climbing apple trees with laughter echoing around her. Despite facing challenges, the Butka family's comfortable home was a haven. Even after the sudden loss of her father, Lily's spirit remained strong. At twelve, she faced a changed world but stood tall, showing a resilience that would define her life.

Her journey from Matatiele to Durban took courage. Leaving home, she found work as a seamstress in a clothing factory, developing skills that would later comfort and support our family. Each piece she made was more than fabric; it was crafted with love and care. I still remember the clothes she made for us, each stitch a symbol of her nurturing spirit.

When she met my father, Spalding, I imagine the spark between them. Their wedding, just days after her 19th birthday, began a new chapter filled with family, laughter, and support. Lily embraced motherhood with unmatched devotion, raising her children while Spalding worked tirelessly to build our dream home. I fondly remember us gathered in my parents' room, saying prayers together. Those moments of faith and closeness tied our family together.

Lily was the nurturing force and the strong guide in our lives. She had a gentle hand but also taught us discipline. I remember the lively chaos of our household — filled with laughter, games, and explorations. When our mischief got out of hand, we faced the consequences, whether it was a scolding or going to bed without dinner. But beneath it all was her deep belief in us, a belief I still carry.

Her kitchen was like a sanctuary, always filled with the aroma of her cooking. She'd pick fresh vegetables and herbs from her garden, turning them into meals that nourished both body and soul. She taught us the importance of sharing, always ensuring there was enough food for anyone who knocked on our door.

As the family grew, Lily became an expert at stretching meals to feed everyone who came by. Dishes like samp and beans, brown stew with dumplings, and frikkadels were staples in our home, each meal a blend of love and resourcefulness. I remember these meals not just for their flavours but for the laughter and stories we shared around the table.

As I grew older, I saw how much of her was in me. Her thriftiness, her fierce love for family, and her strength are all parts of who I am. I see her in how I care for my own children and in the love I pour into every meal. I often draw on her grace and determination as I face the challenges of motherhood.

My mother experienced her own heartache. Losing her son, Elvin, was a grief that deeply affected her, leaving an unforgettable mark on our family. Later, the loss of my father, Spalding, left her to face life alone, a difficult and emotional change.

In her last days, I sensed her strength gently fading. It felt as though she was ready to reunite with the love of her life. I was visiting home in South Africa from London, where I had lived since 2002. This fortunate timing allowed me to say goodbye and for her to meet my twin boys, who were just seven months old.

On July 25, 2009, my mother, Lily Rosalie Trow, passed away suddenly at the age of 79 from a heart attack. Although she's no longer with us, her spirit lives on in my heart. I carry her wisdom, love, and strength with me each day. I feel proud to be her daughter, to have inherited her qualities, and to share her story with the world. Each day, I try to pass down her love to my children, just as she did for me.

Honouring my family's legacy is important to me. The story of the Trow and Butka families is one of resilience, courage, and strength. As I look back on their lives, I feel immense pride and a renewed commitment to carry their legacy forward.

Rochelle Trow

Forging Resilience: A Silent Defence for the Heart

The Silent Forge

In the hushed shadows of my childhood days,

Where laughter danced yet always felt so far,

I learned to weave my heart in muted ways,

Behind a wall of steel, beneath each scar.

At the dinner table, voices swirled and soared,

Yet mine was lost beneath the bustling hum.

Affection felt a distant, fragile chord,

So, I grew quiet, yearning for a crumb of love.

Through windows, I would gaze at worlds outside,

Where siblings thrived, learning to embrace their light.

No one said I couldn't let my true self glide,

Yet no one reached for me, to share that flight.

Awakening to Wholeness

In school, a ghost, I wore the label "rebel,"

Blending in the throng, a shadow in the fray.

Each smallest hurt, though none of them were fatal,

Built a fortress strong, locking pain away.

So, the armour thickened, each layer fortified,

A heart encased in silence, cold as steel,

A child who learned to hide, to never confide,

Belonging felt wrong; revealing seemed unreal.

Now, piece by piece, I'm daring to unveil

The walls I crafted, letting light seep through.

But scars remain, etched deep like a tale,

Whispers of abandonment, of love untrue.

In the quiet forge of memory and pain,

I'm learning to embrace the cracks and flaws.

Each wound a story, each tear a refrain,

A symphony of healing, breaking silent laws.

For in the tender light, I find my voice,

A melody of hope rising from the night.

I'll forge anew, reclaiming by choice,

A heart unbound, embracing love's pure light.

I was the youngest of eleven kids, the final piece in a big, mixed-race family living through apartheid in South Africa. When I was born, my arrival brought the usual happiness that comes with a new baby, but it also added to the heavy load my parents already carried. They had so many struggles, so many mouths to feed, and I often wonder how they managed to find the energy to care for me. How could they love me completely when their hearts were already stretched thin trying to keep the rest of the family safe and fed?

When I think about my early life, I feel both grateful and sad. My parents were focused on keeping us alive in a world that offered very little to families like ours. Their goals were simple: make sure we had food, a roof over our heads, and some safety in a society that seemed stacked against us. They didn't have the luxury to think about our emotional needs. Back then, like many parents of their time, they believed children should be seen but not heard. To them, discipline and silence were virtues. But within that silence, deep, invisible wounds were created — wounds that would affect us all in ways we wouldn't fully understand until much later.

Growing up during apartheid meant I faced racial tensions every day. I was neither black nor white, and that left me in an uncertain, uncomfortable place. The term "coloured" was the label we carried, a reminder of how society saw us — as outsiders, stuck in the middle of an unjust system. I remember feeling the weight of expectations from an early age. Even as a little kid, I noticed the way people looked through me, as if I wasn't there. It made me feel like I didn't belong, and it added to the other burdens I carried. Our home may have protected us from the chaos outside, but it couldn't shield me from the emotional distance I felt from my parents.

I wonder now what it was like for them as parents. They had ten kids to raise, and they were also grieving the loss of our firstborn brother. Losing a child leaves a scar that never really heals. It breaks something inside that others can't see. How could they have had enough love to go around for all of us? I know they loved us, but it didn't always feel like enough. I missed out on little things — the warmth of a hug, a kind word now and then. Instead, there were sharp words, a quick dismissal here or there. These small things may sound trivial, but they left marks on my young heart, creating a quiet kind of pain. Without even realising it, I started to build a wall around myself.

That wall wasn't something I consciously chose to build; it was more of an instinct. It was like a small animal curling up to protect itself. Bit by bit, I began to close off my heart. Every hurtful moment, every time I felt ignored or unseen, added another layer to this emotional armour. I didn't understand it then, but each layer was making it harder for me to trust or to let anyone in. By the time I was grown, I had built walls so thick that they blocked out both the bad and the good. I had closed myself off from experiencing real joy and connection.

In his book "The Untethered Soul," Michael Singer talks about how we shut down in response to pain. He explains that while these walls protect us from hurt, they also keep us from truly living. We miss out on life's beauty, its spontaneity, and the deep relationships that only come from being open to love. Singer encourages us to face our pain, to allow ourselves to feel so that we can begin to tear down these walls. Through my own journey of self-discovery, I've come to see that being vulnerable isn't a weakness; it's actually a strength. It's a door to real, meaningful relationships and a fuller, richer life. Leaning into discomfort is hard, but it's helped me find a way to open my heart again.

Yet, despite everything, there were happy times in my childhood. Our house was sometimes filled with laughter. I can still hear my siblings' voices echoing down the hallway, our shared jokes giving us a break from the heaviness of reality. We had afternoons in the sun, playing games, our laughter floating on the breeze — a small escape from everything else. But those good times couldn't completely erase the feeling of being unseen and unheard. My parents weren't bad people; they were doing their best in a system that wore everyone down. They fought their own battles, and without meaning to, I ended up carrying some of the emotional baggage left behind. Those unintended wounds stayed with me, a shadow I still carry today.

Looking back, I see that my armour was a way to survive in a world that felt harsh and uncertain. But while it protected me, it also kept me from truly living. Learning to take down those walls has been one of the hardest things I've ever done. Each layer I peel away reveals a vulnerable side I had long buried — a tender part of me that feels unfamiliar and a bit scary. The process of healing hasn't been straightforward; it's a winding road with ups and downs, moments of clarity mixed with setbacks. But I'm learning to sit with my own emotions, even the difficult ones.

All these little moments, though they might seem insignificant on their own, added up over time. They formed a pattern of quiet withdrawal, teaching me that it was safer to hide behind my wall than to risk the vulnerability of being truly seen or heard. Feelings of abandonment took root in my heart, and my emotional outbursts became my way of shielding myself from the loneliness that grew within our large family. This struggle gave me independence and pushed me to find my own way, but it also came at a cost.

Now, I want to invite you to join me on a journey. We'll go through some of the most important moments from my childhood and early university years, followed by my time in two different corporate environments in South Africa in the 1990s, both before and after apartheid ended. These experiences may seem ordinary, but together they shaped the armour I built around myself and deepened the wounds that kept me distanced from who I really was. This journey happened against the backdrop of a society filled with pressure, expectations, and constant challenges.

Not all of the armour I built came from pain. Early on, I learned important lessons about leadership that spoke to the kind of person I wanted to become. Strangely, though, I found myself holding onto past hurts and wounds, letting them overshadow those valuable lessons. As I got deeper into my career, I began to set aside the core leadership principles I once valued. Instead, I started to go along with the flow of corporate politics just to survive, and in doing so, I slowly lost sight of who I really was.

Still, even as I dig through these painful memories, I hold onto hope. I believe that healing is possible, and I'm convinced that the journey back to being my true self is worth every step of the way.

Defining Moments: The Events That Shaped My Identity

A Flawed Welcome: My Journey Begins

Being the youngest of eleven children, I often wonder if my arrival was a blessing or a challenge for my family. I was born when my mother was 41, right in the middle of her caring for three very young children. My sister Lavern was just a year old, and my brother Sherwin was only two. With so many kids to feed and care for, our home was always bustling, full of noise, each of us hoping for some of her attention in a crowded household.

My father worked long hours, often far from home, leaving my mother to manage everything on her own with ten kids. It must have been incredibly exhausting, especially as she was also dealing with menopause during our early years. She had already raised seven children before us and now faced the challenge of three more, all needing her in different ways. I sometimes picture her as a ship lost at sea, overwhelmed by waves of responsibility, her sails flapping in the storm of motherhood.

In those early days, life felt chaotic. My siblings and I, especially Sherwin and Lavern, weren't the healthiest children. My mother tried her best to divide her attention, but my older sisters — Jennifer, Marlyn, and Dawn — were either away at boarding school or, when home, busy with college or jobs. Their presence offered brief moments of calm, yet I still felt isolated.

Marlyn, especially, stepped in as a second mother to me. Her laughter filled our home, a comforting sound that helped ease my loneliness. She did her best to comfort me, but my memories of that time are blurry, mostly pieced together from family stories. I was known as the "crazy baby" — a label that, looking back, I think came from my deep need for attention. I'd stand in my crib, gripping the bars, screaming in frustration, and sometimes even scratching my face until it bled. I can't fully explain why I did it, but I think I was simply desperate for a connection that always felt out of reach.

I also had a milk allergy, though it took a while for my family to figure it out. Each painful reaction only added to my distress, creating a cycle of discomfort and confusion. I imagine what it must have felt like as a baby, dealing with a strange, painful feeling in my stomach, crying for relief. But with my mother often busy with my siblings, I spent a lot of time alone in my crib. She didn't want to leave me alone; she just didn't have a choice. During those times, I learned to comfort myself, finding some peace by sucking my thumb and rocking back and forth.

Through this, I learned a hard lesson that would follow me into adulthood: I was alone, and I had to take care of myself. Affection felt foreign to me. Hugs were rare, and I grew up believing that love wasn't something freely given — it was something you had to earn. I moved through life cautiously, never fully trusting that someone would be there to catch me if I fell. I remember longing for a hug, but I never knew how to ask for it, never knew how to express that deep need. So instead, I became independent, convinced that if I just worked hard enough and succeeded, I'd finally earn the love I was missing.

Oprah Winfrey and Dr. Bruce Perry's book *What Happened to You?* deeply resonates with me. They explain how early childhood experiences shape our emotions and how wounds aren't always about violence. Sometimes, they're just the quiet absence of affection that leaves the deepest marks. They say, "When we understand the impact of trauma, we can better support healing for ourselves and others."

Looking back on my childhood, I see that my emotional struggles weren't because of blatant neglect but rather the lack of nurturing that all babies naturally need. I remember watching my nieces and nephews getting hugs and kisses, hearing their laughter fill the room as they soaked up the love around them. Meanwhile, I often felt like an outsider, wondering why those gestures of affection seemed so natural for them but somehow out of reach for me.

This longing for connection left a hole inside me, one I tried to fill by achieving and looking for approval. I put everything into whatever I did, believing that if I could just prove myself, I might finally earn the love I was looking for. But even with these accomplishments, I often felt isolated and not quite good enough, always thinking that I wasn't as worthy of love as others were.

This all ties into what Brené Brown talks about in *The Gifts of Imperfection*, where she says, "Connection is why we're here; it is what gives purpose and meaning to our lives." Back then, I didn't realise that this drive for approval was unhealthy. It pushed me to be successful, but it came at the cost of my own happiness. As I moved through life, I carried these scars without fully understanding how they shaped me.

It wasn't until my late forties that I started to see how my past influenced both my strengths and my struggles. I realised that my relentless push for excellence was really a way to fill the emptiness left by emotional neglect. My drive to prove myself was rooted in a deep fear of being unworthy of love and connection.

Looking back, I now understand that true strength isn't about being independent all the time; it's about being able to be vulnerable and seek connections. Acknowledging my past has been a crucial step in healing, allowing me to reclaim parts of myself that I'd kept buried for so long. Through this journey, I'm slowly learning to reshape my relationship with love, both for myself and for others.

Becoming an Aunt at Five: Witnessing Love I Never Knew

My oldest sister, Jennifer, was twenty years older than me, and I had seen my other siblings begin their adult lives. But nothing could prepare me for how much things would change with the arrival of my niece and nephew. Jennifer's wedding was a blur of bright colours and happy laughter. I was only five years old, just a small figure in the background, swept up in the excitement but too young to really understand what was happening. What stood out to me most was how everyone came together for her, showering her with love and blessings. It was beautiful and left a mark on me.

What truly changed everything, though, was when my sister Dawn had her daughter, Melanie. Suddenly, I was an aunt. There was a new baby in the house, and everything felt different. Melanie was tiny, wrapped in soft pink blankets, with little fingers that curled and uncurled as she slept. I was fascinated by her, but at the same time, I felt something I didn't quite understand: jealousy. The attention that used to be mine now felt split, and I didn't know how to handle it.

Not long after, my sister Merle, who lived in Cape Town, came home with her son, Marc. I was both excited and jealous again. At such a young age, I didn't have the words to explain my feelings. It felt like I was being pushed aside in my own family. Everyone seemed so focused on the babies that I didn't know where I fit anymore.

I watched my mom hold Melanie and Marc with a tenderness I couldn't remember experiencing myself. The way she cradled them, her arms steady and full of love, was something I longed for but didn't know how to ask for. I felt like I was on the outside looking in, watching a kind of love I hadn't been given. My mom wasn't cold or unloving; she had been overwhelmed when I was born. But as a child, I couldn't understand that. All I knew was that I wanted what Melanie and Marc had—someone's undivided love and attention.

To get attention, I acted out. I'd take Melanie outside, pretending to help her, but then I'd drink from her bottle myself. I didn't care if anyone noticed me being mischievous as long as I wasn't invisible. I just wanted my mom or someone else to look at me the way they looked at the babies. My sister Dawn likes to remind me of how I used to sneak snacks from Melanie's lunchbox when we went to school together. I thought her food was better than mine, so I'd wait for the right moment to steal a treat. I didn't think about Melanie missing her lunch; I just wanted something that made me feel special, even if it was just a tastier sandwich.

My older siblings thought I was rude and difficult, but I don't think they understood why. I wasn't trying to be mean or bad. I was just a little girl who wanted to feel loved and noticed. When I was with my siblings, I'd cling to my dad and say, "He's my father, not yours!" I wanted to make it clear that he was mine, as if saying it out loud would make me feel less left out.

At home, when my mom went shopping, she'd lock us inside the house for safety. But I figured out how to climb through the window to escape and play with my friends. I'd stay out as long as I could, watching for my mom's figure climbing up the street. As soon as I saw her, I'd hurry back inside, pretending I'd been there the whole time. I loved those moments of freedom—running around with my friends and feeling like I belonged somewhere. Even if it was brief, it gave me a sense of joy I couldn't find at home.

School wasn't much easier. My sister Marlyn, who was like a second mom to me, was also my first-grade teacher. I told everyone she was my real mom and said my actual mom was my grandmother because she seemed so much older than other kids' parents. Marlyn was the one who came to school meetings and stepped in when I got into trouble. She filled the gaps my mom couldn't, but even then, I felt like I was constantly seeking approval. I was always getting into mischief, not to be mean but because I wanted someone to notice me.

Brené Brown once wrote, "Vulnerability is the birthplace of innovation, creativity, and change." Looking back, I think I was too young to understand vulnerability or what I was really feeling. I thought I had to compete for love and attention. Instead of real connection, I thought love was something you had to fight for.

When I reflect on those early years, I now see that love was all around me, just in ways I didn't understand then. Love isn't always about who gets the most hugs or attention. Sometimes it's about the chaos of a big family and the quiet moments of connection that sneak in between the noise. But as a child, I misunderstood it all. I thought I wasn't loved enough, and that belief shaped how I viewed myself and my relationships for years.

As I got older, especially in my late forties, I began to untangle these feelings. I realised my mischief and jealousy weren't just about wanting attention; they were about wanting to feel worthy of love. I now know that love doesn't have to be earned—it's something we all deserve. And while those early years were filled with confusion and longing, they also taught me the power of connection and the importance of being open to love, even when it looks different than what I expected.

Books as an Escape: Embracing Avoidance and Fantasy

As a child, I found comfort in books, tucking myself into a quiet corner of the room I shared with three or four others, like a moth drawn to a flame. I would borrow books from the public library— not just one, but whole stacks— each book a ticket to another world, far from the limits of my reality. I can still picture myself standing in the library, looking at the shelves and wondering, "What will I read next?" That thrill of discovery often came with a bit of anxiety, a worry that I'd eventually run out of stories to lose myself in.

Reading wasn't just a hobby; it was my escape. My mother had a strict bedtime schedule, believing in order above all, so I would sneak a flashlight under my blankets to keep reading late into the night. The night shadows would wrap around me, but in my books, I was free. At the sound of footsteps, I'd quickly hide the light and pretend to sleep. My heart would race with both excitement and fear— a small act of rebellion that felt necessary.

When my brother Alvin came home, he often brought chaos with him. Back then, I didn't understand that he was struggling with his own battles, using alcohol to cope. I only felt his anger and the fear his outbursts spread through our home. My mother, who I later understood was trying to protect us, often sent us away while she faced his anger alone. Her acceptance of his behaviour showed her love, though I didn't see it that way back then.

In those scary moments, I turned to my books—not just as an escape but as a shield against a reality that felt too heavy. I remember crawling under my bed, clutching a book to my chest, the words blurring as I held back tears. In a way, my safe place became a crutch, a way to block out the storm around me. As I grew older, I realised this habit had left a mark on me, teaching me to push down my feelings instead of facing them—a lesson learned in the shadows of my childhood.

Looking back, I see how this habit of avoiding things shaped me as an adult. I carried it into my marriage, ignoring problems and convincing myself that staying quiet was easier than speaking up. But this only allowed issues to grow and eventually led to our breakup. By avoiding vulnerability, I missed the chance for deeper connections and growth in my life.

This was a tough lesson. What once gave me comfort—the fantasy in books—had become a wall that kept me from truly living and feeling. It was like a ship in a storm, choosing to sail away from the waves instead of facing them.

Everything changed when my twin sons were born. Suddenly, I felt a love so strong it shook my whole being. Yet I realised that I still struggled to communicate this love. My old patterns of avoiding emotions were now affecting my children. Determined to change, we started a journey of healing together. We sought help, worked with coaches, and learned to express our feelings, sharing love and frustrations in ways that built connections rather than barriers. Watching my sons grow, I feel proud of how well they communicate, a testament to the work we've done together.

As Brené Brown says in her book *Daring Greatly*, "We don't have to do it all alone. We were never meant to." For much of my life, I turned to books to escape from the loneliness that coloured my reality. Now, as I reclaim my story, I see that real connections come not from avoiding but from embracing vulnerability and honesty. This path hasn't been easy, but it has shown me the way toward a life with emotional balance and authenticity, guiding me to embrace my true self and build stronger relationships.

Looking to the future, I feel a deep sense of hope. I want my sons to find their own way, equipped with the wisdom and resilience that I struggled to gain. I picture them engaging with the world wholeheartedly, stepping into the light instead of retreating into shadows of doubt or fear.

The power of stories has guided me, and now I'm determined to shape my own. I welcome the ups and downs of life rather than hiding from them. Each twist in my journey is a lesson, a stepping stone for my sons as they walk their own paths.

In this new chapter, I aim to show them the courage to face adversity, the empathy to connect with others, and the curiosity to explore all life offers. Together, we celebrate the beauty of vulnerability and the strength in being real. I hope they carry forward not only my dreams for them but also their own, free from the limitations I once felt bound by.

The Weight of Unintentional Labels: Growing Shame

Growing up in the Trow family felt like moving through a maze, where every turn came with expectations and unspoken rules. Every moment drew me deeper into a world where labels stuck to me, hard to shake off. My mother, a devoted Catholic, found comfort in her faith rituals. As the youngest, I was expected to follow her lead, keeping step with the rhythm of prayers and confessions. To her, the church was sacred, and I was her child soldier, wearing the armour of belief, even when it felt uncomfortable and heavy.

I can still remember those Saturdays spent in the confessional, the smell of polished wood and incense wrapping around me like a blanket. But as a kid, what did I really have to confess? I was just a child trying to make sense of a world that already saw me as flawed. Often, I'd lie about attending confession, choosing freedom over the discomfort of judgmental eyes. It was easier to avoid than to explain why these "sacred" rituals felt more like a burden than a comfort.

Lent and Christmas became grand displays of our family's faith, where expectations felt heavier than the events themselves. Kneeling beside my mother's bed during Lent to say the rosary felt more like a chore than a spiritual journey, a role I played without meaning. I wanted to understand my beliefs without the weight of dogma that shaped our household. Instead, I rebelled against the foundations laid for me. The more I pushed back, the deeper the shame rooted itself, making me question not only my faith but also my self-worth.

This shame didn't stop with religion; it crept into other areas, especially in my mixed-race family. Hair and body became constant battlegrounds, with my sisters critiquing each curl and every inch of our bodies. Growing up in apartheid-era South Africa, where race and appearance pressures were intense, their comments stung. "Neaten it up" became a regular instruction, pushing me to fit their idea of beauty, ideals that felt wrong for me. Why was straight hair the "right" look? I longed to embrace my own beauty, which felt like a quiet defiance against the norms around me.

Body shaming was a familiar voice at every family gathering, each event turning into a stage for hurtful observations. "Oh, you've put on weight" was a common remark, hitting my confidence as if it were casual instead of a sharp blow. Comparing myself to siblings and friends only deepened my sense of being "less than." I was the rebel, the outcast, always in trouble, told I could be better but never really knowing how to break free.

At school, acceptance felt like an urgent need. I remember sneaking into the bathroom to smoke—not because I wanted to but because it was what the "cool" kids did. I craved acceptance, a way to throw off the shame that had been hanging over me. My first boyfriend was another attempt to fit in, a relationship that added nothing but gave me a moment to feel like I belonged.

Each act of rebellion, every wrong choice, was an effort to find myself in a world set on defining me by what I was not. The shame of feeling not enough, of constant comparison, followed me, keeping me tied to a past I wanted to escape.

Reflecting now, I realise that finding self-acceptance has been a long journey, marked by challenges that tested me but also helped me break free from the weight of labels. Each step has been filled with moments of reflection, where the shame of the past flickered, reminding me of battles fought against expectations. By embracing our imperfections—those scars we often hide—we can build real connections and find a place in a world that can feel lonely.

Brené Brown says in *Daring Greatly* that facing our vulnerabilities lets us break the chains of shame, turning it into a source of strength. This change lets us rise from insecurity and step into our real selves. True courage isn't about being perfect but being willing to be seen, to step into life openly and share our stories—the good and the tough. Every story, no matter how messy, can heal—not just ourselves but others who connect with it. In shared vulnerability, we create a richer human experience, full of empathy and understanding.

Now, as a mother, I take on the role of guiding my children as they find their own paths. I teach them to appreciate their natural beauty, to value their uniqueness, and to choose their own beliefs and spirituality. I give them different perspectives, trusting that they'll find what resonates in their hearts. This not only supports their independence but also lets me redefine my own relationship with faith, becoming clearer on my spirituality.

My faith now centres on a personal relationship with God, found in quiet moments of reflection and gratitude rather than the limits of organised religion. This direct connection gives me peace and strength in my beliefs, helping me understand my place in the universe. With each step, I see that every challenge, every moment of vulnerability, brings me closer to understanding myself and to creating a legacy of authenticity for my children. Together, we build a space where they can explore who they are, question norms, and ultimately grow into strong, empowered individuals, free from the labels that once tried to define us.

Curiosity Misunderstood: Labelled as Rebellion in School

When I think about my school years, they seem like a distant blur, a time when excitement was rare. The way we were taught was strict and dull, filled with dry facts that never captured my curiosity. I often felt stuck in a routine of textbooks, wishing for more engaging discussions. Every time I raised my hand to ask questions, hoping to learn more, I was often scolded. "You're being disruptive," they would say, as if wanting to know more was a bad thing.

There wasn't much encouragement, and the subjects I could study further were decided based on my past performance. But that performance wasn't always about my abilities—it was often due to a teaching style that didn't suit me. Somehow, I got through school. But now, looking back, I realise I was like a fish out of water. I learn best by hearing and doing, and the rigid way we were taught didn't match how I think and absorb knowledge. Teachers rarely went the extra mile, so we learned to memorise instead of really understanding and sharpening our thinking skills. I've come to realise that this reflective nature is just who I am, which explains why I always felt out of place.

One memory still stands out—a teacher told me I wouldn't amount to anything if I didn't change my behaviour. I remember feeling a rush of defiance. That moment stayed with me for years. Looking back, I know the teacher wasn't trying to hurt me, but their words sparked something deep inside. I thought to myself, "I'll show you. I will become something." Those words became my unlikely motivation, pushing me to work hard and aim high, even if it meant going against the grain.

When it was time to think about my future, my mom suggested I become a teacher or a nurse—safe jobs with financial support available. But the rebel in me didn't like that idea. "I'm going to university to become a lawyer," I told her firmly, even though I had no idea how I'd pay for it. To make her happy, I applied to teacher's college too, but deep down, I knew I wouldn't end up in a classroom.

At a key point in my decision-making, my mom sent me on a vacation to Cape Town to visit my sister Merle and her husband, Curm, who was a high school principal. She hoped the trip would give me time to figure things out. In Cape Town, surrounded by beauty, I started feeling more confident. I had a part-time job, which gave me a taste of independence and some financial help for university. I started believing I could make it work somehow.

My rebellious spirit thrived on challenges. That feeling of being different, combined with the shame I sometimes felt, pushed me to create my own path. Strangely, I owe some of that drive to the teacher who doubted me. Their harsh words lit a fire in me, making me determined to succeed. But I didn't realise back then that this drive would also pull me away from the person I truly wanted to be.

This intense need to excel came at a price. While it helped me build a successful career, it also made me feel like I always had something to prove. I wasn't satisfied, constantly chasing perfection. This led to an unhealthy pattern of overworking, sacrificing relationships, and neglecting my well-being just to climb the corporate ladder and earn recognition.

Now, I see that my so-called rebellious spirit, which came from my curiosity and misunderstood ambitions, became both my biggest strength and my heaviest burden. The good part is that I've started learning the importance of balance—a lesson I'm still working on every day.

As a mom, I want my kids to have the best education possible. That's why my top financial priority has always been their private school fees. I believe that with good values and the right support, this kind of education can help them build on their strengths and focus on happiness instead of society's often warped ideas of success.

I want my kids to grow up in a world where their curiosity is welcomed and encouraged. A world that builds on their strengths rather than pushing them to fix areas they don't enjoy or struggle with. I want them to have the confidence to believe there's enough in the world for everyone, without constant competition or pressure to meet society's unnecessary demands for respect.

Embracing Failure: A Pivotal Moment of Acceptance

I remember the first time I felt the heavy weight of expectations. My parents, though supportive of my decision to attend university, didn't have the money or experience to guide me through choosing a career. I had to figure it out on my own, which was tough for someone still learning to find their way.

The voice of my high school teacher still rings in my ears: "You'll amount to nothing if you don't change your behaviour." I promised myself, "I'll show you," and that promise drove me to work harder than ever. Back in 1989, it was rare for someone from a coloured high school to go to university. It was during the last years of apartheid in South Africa, and though white universities had started to open their doors to people of colour, the process was far from easy. Going to university was my first big step in proving the doubters wrong.

Becoming the first in my family to go to university felt huge. My parents were proud but also worried. I had to borrow money from my sister for tuition, and I knew they feared I might fail because of my so-called rebellious nature. Now, I understand their concerns better. Paying for my education taught me to value money and how to make sacrifices—lessons that have stayed with me.

With independence came my tendency to take on too much, something I've done throughout my life. I balanced full-time classes, a part-time job, and an active social life, often going out to clubs with friends on weekends. It was exciting but exhausting, and it set a pattern for how I approached life. Being a coloured student at a mostly white university during apartheid made me feel like an outsider. But I found comfort in friendships that crossed racial lines, showing me that deep down, we all want to be accepted and understood.

At university, I faced failures that felt overwhelming. I remember failing a semester course because my last-minute cramming wasn't enough. Those moments forced me to realise I needed a better approach. I started focusing on understanding the material instead of just passing.

Looking back at my time in a coloured school, I see how unprepared I was for university. My education was nowhere near as strong as that of my white peers, who had better resources and opportunities. Starting university in 1989, as South Africa was on the brink of change, I joined political protests for equality. It took five more years for apartheid to end, and even today, the effects are still felt.

The biggest failure came when I realised I wasn't cut out to be a lawyer. I had gone to university determined to pursue law, but I didn't understand what it really involved. The endless case studies and detailed laws felt suffocating, and my creative side struggled. Admitting that law wasn't for me was a turning point. It taught me that changing direction isn't a weakness—it's a sign of self-awareness. But back then, I saw it as a failure and carried a lot of shame for not achieving what I set out to do. In the end, I graduated with a Bachelor of Social Science degree and left my dream of law behind.

After graduating, I joined a well-known retailer, a company that had supported me through school and university. Their Retail Management Program felt like a fresh start—a chance to leave my shame behind and prove myself to my parents.

In this new role, I learned the importance of being flexible. I realised that one setback doesn't mean the end of everything. Instead, each failure taught me a lesson and helped me grow. But it wasn't always easy. I often found myself being too hard on myself, questioning why I wasn't good enough.

Looking back now, I see that those failures weren't just obstacles—they were essential parts of my journey. Failing doesn't mean giving up. It means finding the courage to try again. Every experience of doubt and every challenge has shaped who I am today. I've learned to accept my failures and see them as stepping stones, not roadblocks. It's this acceptance that has kept me moving forward, even when my ego was bruised. Embracing failure has been a key part of becoming who I am and learning to start over when needed.

Navigating the Workforce During Apartheid: A Challenging Entry

I still remember the day Charles, a manager at the store where I worked, saw something in me that I hadn't yet seen in myself. It was a quiet but life-changing moment. He invited me to join the company's Retail Management Trainee program. That opportunity was a turning point in my career, and I've always been deeply grateful for it.

In that program, I was introduced to Stephen Covey's book *The Seven Habits of Highly Effective People*. Those lessons became a big part of my personal and professional growth. I loved learning about being proactive, setting priorities, and communicating effectively. These weren't just theories to me—they were tools I could use every day. That experience sparked a passion for continuous learning and self-improvement, something I carry with me even now.

The program also made me believe in myself and understand the kind of leader I wanted to be. I learned that leadership isn't about being perfect; it's about growing, helping others, and making a positive impact.

But my time at this retail company also showed me the hard realities of working during apartheid. Even though South Africa was moving toward democracy, the workplace still carried old habits and attitudes. I heard offhand comments and saw behaviours that were clear reminders of the past.

The corporate world also had its own challenges. It was competitive, and some people were willing to step on others to get ahead. I was part of a very small group of people of colour in the Retail Management Program—just one African, one Indian, and me, a Coloured person. Most of our colleagues were white. It often felt like we were there just to tick a box, rather than because of our skills or potential. This made it clear how much work was still needed to make real change.

Despite this, I learned an important lesson early on: success doesn't have to come at the expense of others. There's room for everyone to do well. I realised that building diverse teams, where people bring different strengths and perspectives, makes everyone stronger. This became one of my core beliefs as a leader: *Together, we're stronger.*

I carried these lessons with me as I grew in my career. I worked hard to create spaces where everyone felt included and valued. For me, this was more than just a professional goal; it was deeply personal. I hated the inequality I saw during apartheid, and it fuelled my desire to create workplaces where everyone had a fair chance to succeed.

I'll never forget working with Jabulani, the security guard at my store in Port Elizabeth. I helped him grow into a salesperson, and eventually, he became a Store Manager and later a District Director overseeing multiple stores in the Western Cape. Watching him succeed brought me so much joy. Moments like that reminded me why I was committed to driving change. I'll always treasure the memory of voting for the first time in early 1994—it was a symbol of hope for a better future.

Still, the challenges didn't disappear. I faced moments that reminded me of the inequalities that lingered. One manager called me a "rough diamond," meaning my work was good, but my communication needed polishing. It stung because I knew I hadn't had the same educational opportunities as some of my colleagues. I couldn't help but wonder if the feedback would have been different if I'd had access to better schooling.

Even with these struggles, I built strong relationships with my teams. I wasn't the kind of leader who stayed distant—I worked alongside them, showing what needed to be done. I valued constructive feedback, but it was frustrating when comments focused on my "rough edges" rather than recognising my effort and dedication.

Eventually, I joined one of the largest and most recognised FMCG (Fast Moving Consumer Goods) companies as a Change Manager, leading a huge IT project that unified South African businesses onto one platform. Kim, the HR Director, saw my potential and hired me even though I didn't have an HR background. That decision changed my life. I found my passion in HR and started building my career in that field.

One of the most memorable experiences under Kim's leadership was a team-building session based on Robert Fulghum's book, *All I Really Need to Know I Learned in Kindergarten.* Even though I never went to kindergarten, the lessons—about sharing, fairness, and kindness—struck a chord with me.

During that session, I realised how important empathy and collaboration are. The activities helped me see gaps in my understanding of teamwork. I learned that vulnerability can bring people closer and that taking time to reflect on my actions is essential. These lessons weren't just useful at work—they became guiding principles in my life.

But I also noticed that the lessons we discussed didn't always translate into actions. For people of colour, there were still subtle but painful reminders of inequality. Sometimes, my fear of failure and rejection overshadowed what I'd learned about leadership. In high-pressure environments, the instinct to survive often took over.

At my new company, I faced similar challenges. I was praised for my work but told I needed to refine my leadership style. It was another reminder that systemic biases still shaped how people saw me, no matter how hard I worked. This pushed me to fight even harder for fairness and to create environments where everyone's contributions were valued.

My time with the South African HR operations team was short, but it led to a promotion to Learning Manager. I created a Finance Academy for South Africa, which raised my profile and opened the door to a role in the company's London Head Office. Being recognised for my work, not my skin colour, was a surreal experience.

In London, I felt like a new chapter had begun. I worked with amazing people, and my mentor, Paul, believed in me and helped me thrive. For the first time, I was in a place where my skills were celebrated, and I didn't feel held back by outdated stereotypes.

Looking back, I see how much those early experiences shaped me. They taught me that leadership is about lifting others up and creating spaces where everyone can succeed. As Maya Angelou said, *"People will forget what you said, people will forget what you did, but people will never forget how you made them feel."* This quote reminds me of the importance of making people feel valued, and it continues to inspire me in everything I do.

In Conclusion

As I wrap up this chapter, I find myself looking back with a mix of emotions—both sadness and hope. *"Forging Armour: A Heart's Silent Defence"* has been a journey of facing challenges and finding strength in vulnerability. For a long time, I held onto the pain and wound I had gone through, thinking they were part of who I was. In doing so, I lost sight of the young leader I wanted to be in South Africa's corporate world.

For 20 years, I built a version of myself that wasn't true to who I really am. As a child, I experienced things I couldn't fully understand or explain, and I didn't have the tools to deal with them. Those moments, small as they seemed back then, stayed with me and shaped how I saw myself. I carried the pain silently, believing it was part of my identity. What I didn't know was that facing these feelings would be the first step to setting myself free.

Looking back, I can now see how much of my past was shaped by these unspoken struggles. It's taken me a long time to realise that I wasn't to blame for what happened to me. I was just a child trying to find my way in a confusing world. I've learned to tell myself that I didn't do anything wrong. I deserved love, kindness, and respect then, just as much as I do now.

This journey of healing hasn't been easy, but it has been deeply important. It's not just about working through things in therapy—it's about healing in every part of who I am, including my heart and soul. It has taken years, but slowly, I'm letting light and love replace the pain.

Standing here now, I feel grateful for how far I've come. Every challenge has taught me something about kindness, compassion, and what it means to be a leader. These values were hidden behind my pain for so long, but now they guide me forward.

This chapter of my life in South Africa, with all its highs and lows, has been full of lessons and meaningful connections. As I prepare for the next stage of my journey, first in London and then in Switzerland, I feel ready to take on new opportunities. These places will be a fresh start, and I'm bringing with me the strength I've built and the lessons I've learned.

With every word I share, I hope to encourage others to face their own struggles, to find strength in being open and vulnerable, and to celebrate the unique stories that make them who they are. This is not the end of my journey—it's just the next step. I'm moving forward, knowing that my pain does not define me. What defines me is my ability to rise above it, to love, and to keep growing.

The Turning Point: Awakening through Awareness

Crossing the Threshold: Closing a Chapter

In the depths of my soul, a storm rages on,

Twenty years of love, now shrouded in dawn.

Deception's veil, a cruel disguise,

Shattering trust, beneath tearful skies.

Each memory tainted, every laugh stained,

The foundation we built, now bruised and strained.

Twenty years of hopes, now shattered dreams,

Lost in a maze of lies and schemes.

Pain so deep, it cuts to the core,

Betrayal's sting, like never before.

How do I heal from this profound ache,

When the love I knew was simply fake?

But through this darkness, I'll find my light,

Strength in my heart, to stand and fight.

For the truth may hurt, but it sets me free,

To reclaim myself and rise, just me.

Yet the decision weighs heavy, a burden to bear,

Each path I envision, a jumble of despair.

Memories flood in, both bitter and sweet,

Echoes of laughter, now bittersweet.

Can I let go of the life we once shared?

The dreams we painted, the moments we dared?

I linger in shadows, where hope used to glow,

Now haunted by whispers of what I must know.

The faces of children, the ties that still bind,

The love that was real, now feels so confined.

How do I choose when my heart's in a bind?

To sever the ties, or seek what's been blind?

Days turn to nights, as I wrestle my fate,

The weight of this choice, an insufferable weight.

But in quiet reflection, I search for my truth,

In the ruins of love, I reclaim my youth.

And though fear grips my heart, a tumultuous tide,

I know in my spirit, I cannot abide.

For the life that I seek cannot thrive in a lie,

I must gather my courage, and learn how to fly.

So I stand at the crossroads, the future unclear,

With the echoes of love, now mixed with my fear.

Yet deep in my heart, a flicker ignites,

A vision of freedom, breaking the nights.

I'll honour the past, but embrace what's to come,

For the strength that I seek is already begun.

In the depths of my soul, amidst storms and despair,

I'll rise from the ashes, my spirit laid bare.

Who could have guessed that our move to Switzerland in 2019 would shake up our lives in ways we never expected? When I started my new job on September 1, 2019, I thought it would just be an exciting career move. Travelling between Switzerland and London every week seemed doable—until it wasn't. This chapter reflects my life as I've experienced it through my unique emotional lens. While I acknowledge that others may remember certain moments differently, I want to share my journey with all its layers and shades, as it is my story.

Weeks turned into months, and every flight made me feel the growing distance from my family. Weekends at home felt far too short, slipping away like sand through my fingers. I was trying to balance work calls, living alone in Zurich—which felt strange and isolating—and managing the boys' au pair schedule from afar. It was overwhelming. Spending four nights a week in hotel rooms or my Zurich apartment blurred the line between work and home, and the routine became suffocating. Then, in March 2020, everything changed. COVID-19 hit like a storm, and suddenly I felt both anxious and relieved. The idea of not boarding another plane for a while brought a strange sense of peace.

For the next three months, I was stuck at home, spending more time with my husband than I ever had before. It felt like the first time we'd been in the same space for so long, but it wasn't as comforting as I'd hoped. COVID didn't create problems in our marriage—it just brought old ones to the surface. Emmett had been once again unemployed and struggling to find a new role. This seemed to be a regular pattern since we left South Africa, and this time, the weight of it felt even heavier. I thought the lockdown might give us a chance to reconnect as a family, but it didn't work out that way. In our London home, Emmett would spend most of the day relaxing while I juggled teleconferences, home schooling the boys, and hunting for groceries in what felt like a daily survival game. I was also worrying about the boys' upcoming move to Swiss schools, the reality of having no support to tackle the unpacked furniture and boxes when we arrived in Zurich at the end of June, and the constant uncertainty of not knowing whether our move would happen or not hanging over us.

Every night, my mind raced with worry. Emmett's late nights and loud snoring often sent me to the spare room just to get some sleep. I was carrying the family's chaos on my shoulders, but instead of seeing it as me trying to hold things together, Emmett dismissed it as me being controlling and worrying about nothing.

In June 2020, the family finally moved to Switzerland to join me. I felt excitement and dread when we arrived at our new home. The boys, then eleven, were upset about leaving London and made sure I knew it, often voicing their frustrations. Their complaints became a regular background noise, reminding me of how much we'd been through. The unpacking process didn't make things any easier. We dealt with damaged furniture and endless boxes, and I felt the stress building as Emmett seemed disengaged from it all. When it came to buying new furniture, it wasn't Emmett who stepped up—it was my niece's husband, Faiek, who helped me out.

Those first few months in Switzerland were some of the hardest in my life. I felt lost in a new country, weighed down by responsibilities that seemed to grow every day. But even in the middle of all this chaos, I learned something valuable. I discovered resilience, found strength in being vulnerable, and learned to ask for help from unexpected places. Looking back, I see that the move wasn't just about starting over in a new country. It was about redefining our family, facing our fears, and uncovering new ways to love and support each other. The road ahead was still uncertain but I was reassured knowing that we were all in it together. But there was a gradual, sinking realisation that perhaps it wasn't entirely true. That things were slowly starting to fall apart.

The Day Everything Changed

I woke up around 5:58 in the morning, feeling the weight of a restless night. The bed felt far too big without Emmett beside me. My mind was racing, trying to figure out what I'd tell the boys when they woke up and asked where their dad was. Lying there in the silence, I felt overwhelmed by worry. By 6:32, I couldn't take it anymore. My fingers trembled as I typed out a message to Emmett: **"What should I tell the kids?"**

Just as I sent the text, Tyson walked into the bedroom. His small frame climbed onto the bed, and he gently stroked my hand, a familiar gesture that usually brought me peace. Moments later, Zach joined us, and for a short while, we lay together, surrounded by warmth and love. Strangely, they didn't ask about their dad. After a while, they got restless and headed downstairs, leaving me alone with my swirling thoughts.

At 7:39, Emmett's loud voice echoed through the house. Hearing him again should've been a relief, but instead, it filled me with dread. Assuming he was drunk, I jumped in the shower, hoping the water would calm my nerves. But the shouting got louder. Then I heard Zach's voice, shaking with fear as he called out, **"Mom, please come down! I think Dad is being silly!"** I told him I'd be right there, but my stomach churned.

When I finally went downstairs to the boys' playroom, I saw Emmett slumped on the sofa. His friend was pacing angrily. Both of them were clearly drunk. Unsure of what to do, I hesitated, then decided to busy myself making a Nespresso lungo. My hands shook as I listened to his friend yelling, his voice filled with rage. He hurled accusations at Emmett, each one sharper than the last. Emmett, meanwhile, just laughed, oblivious to the tension.

Things quickly escalated. His friend's anger boiled over as he shouted about Emmett's behaviour. Each accusation he hurled at Emmett felt like a stab in my heart, as I was most disappointed by what I was hearing, knowing that there was truth to his words. I wanted all the loud voices to stop it as the children were becoming increasingly anxious about the two drunken men's behaviour, to pull Emmett out of his drunken haze, but fear kept me frozen.

Then chaos erupted. Emmett, fuelled by anger, stood up and threw his friend and his suitcase out into the street. The boys started crying, their terrified voices cutting through the madness. My instincts took over. I grabbed their hands and ushered them back into the house. **"Go upstairs, stay there!"** I whispered urgently, my voice trembling as I tried to shield them from the scene.

When I turned back, Emmett's furious eyes locked on mine. He screamed at me, blaming me for everything. His face was twisted with anger. My heart raced as I tried to block his flailing arms. I felt powerless, so small. All I wanted was to protect the boys from seeing this side of their father that appeared in when he was badgered in a drunken rage.

Before long, the doorbell rang. My stomach dropped—I knew it was the police as I heard his friend telling a neighbour he called the police. Emmett brushed past me, leaning in close and hissing through clenched teeth, **"Stand your ground. Don't you dare take his side."** I was trembling but forced myself to answer the door.

Two male officers stepped inside. Their serious expressions added to my unease. I tried to explain the situation, saying Emmett and his friend had come home drunk and were now fighting. My words felt heavy, like they weren't enough to convey the chaos that had just unfolded. The officers turned to Emmett, who tried to act composed but was clearly unsteady on his feet. Standing back, I watched in disbelief as he lied to them, painting a picture far removed from the truth. Eventually, the police decided to leave, saying they'd call Emmett on Monday to arrange a time for him to come in sober, possibly with a translator. I nodded and thanked them as I showed them out.

When I went back inside, the house was eerily quiet. Emmett had gone upstairs to sleep, leaving an oppressive stillness behind. My thoughts immediately turned to the boys. I found them huddled together in one of their rooms. Their eyes were wide with fear and confusion. They asked me what was going to happen as they knew the police had come, and my heart broke. **"Dad's asleep now,"** I reassured them softly. **"Everything's fine."**

But it wasn't fine. That day, the events replayed in my head over and over like a broken record. Each time, they brought fresh pain as I recalled the accusations of his friends, which I knew within my heart were true. Emmett's reckless behaviour stung deeply. I kept asking myself why. Why would he do this? Was I not enough? The questions consumed me, twisting in my stomach like a knife. I felt like a robot moving through the weekend. I kept things as normal as I could for the boys—making their meals, playing games, and keeping them busy. But inside, I was falling apart. I had no one to turn to for support, not in this new country. I felt completely alone. On Sunday, Emmett sent me an email apologising. I read it over and over, looking for something that could ease the turmoil inside me. But his words felt hollow, like they were just there to cover up his guilt.

I thought back to all the times I'd ignored the signs—the late nights, the excuses, the dishevelled look when he came home. I wanted to believe in him, but now I wasn't sure if I'd been blind to the truth all along. Looking back, I saw a pattern. Emmett seemed to thrive on control and power. His drive to succeed had once seemed like a positive trait, but now it felt like the thing pulling us apart. I'd grown, evolved, while he seemed stuck in the past, living in a fantasy of his own making. I sat there, overwhelmed by the heartbreaking realisation: the man I once adored had become a stranger.

Reflections on Our Marriage: The Journey to My Decision to Divorce

In the months that followed, I poured my heart into my journal. Writing felt like having an honest conversation with Emmett, but even when I shared some of it with him, it felt like my words vanished into thin air, never truly reaching him. Thinking about our marriage stirs up so many emotions—sadness, frustration, and a deep sense of loss. It's clear we've come to a turning point, one we both seem too afraid to face. His recent behaviour has brought up old wounds and highlighted how unhappy I've been for so long. It feels like he expects me to overlook his flaws and put my own needs aside, as though it's my duty as his wife to make sacrifices.

I've seen women in his family push their desires and happiness to the background, and I feel stuck in that same story. But I can't keep living like this. It's heartbreaking to realise that his idea of being the "alpha male" seems to come at the cost of my happiness and identity. I used to think marriage was about partnership—about supporting and adapting to each other. But I've given up so much of myself just to avoid fights and keep the peace.

The cracks in our relationship grew even wider after our twin boys were born in 2008. It felt like he wanted me to stay the same reliable partner while ignoring how much our lives had changed. I tried to tell him, over and over, that I needed more support, but he never seemed to listen. He brushed off my concerns as small complaints and never stopped to think about why I was so desperate for help. Over time, I became more and more frustrated, but he stayed the same, wrapped up in his routines, while I felt like I was disappearing.

After nearly 20 years of marriage, I feel like I'm only valued for what I do to meet his expectations. It's devastating to think that even though we've built a life that looks successful from the outside—careers, financial stability—I still feel emotionally empty. He tells me he loves me, but his actions don't back up those words. Love isn't enough; I need respect. Without that respect, our marriage is falling apart. The trust we once had is gone. I can't count on him to keep his promises, big or small. It feels like he's living in his own world, where his needs and wants come first. He's kind and generous to everyone outside our home, but at home, I feel unappreciated and overlooked.

It's shocking how far apart we've grown. Sitting here in Switzerland, I keep replaying that Saturday morning in my mind. That moment—when I felt truly unsafe—was a turning point. Instead of calming my fears, he exploded in anger, even in front of our children. I can still see the rage in his eyes as he threw his friend out of the house, ripping his sweater in the process. He turned that anger on me too, screaming like a man out of control. How could I possibly feel safe after that? It wasn't just that one moment. He's yelled at me with the same intensity, whether sober or drunk, over the years. I've tried to tell him how his anger makes me feel, but he just gets defensive, accusing me of exaggerating. It's exhausting to live like this, always on edge, never knowing what might set him off. While he's never physically hurt me, the fear and tension are always there.

After all these years, I don't even recognise the person I've become. I've worked so hard to break the patterns of my past—to be better than the mother who lashed out when she was overwhelmed. But now, I feel like I'm turning into her. I snap at the smallest things, and I hate it. At work, I'm respected and valued. At home, I feel invisible. He was supposed to be the one person who really understood me. But over time, he's changed. He's become more self-absorbed, refusing to see what's right in front of him. His constant half-truths have made me feel like I've lost my own integrity just by being around him. I can't reconcile the man he is now with the man I fell in love with.

I think back to the speech I gave at his 50th birthday in October 2019. I poured so much into those words because I knew how disappointed he was with what I said at his 40th. I wanted it to be perfect. I thanked him for believing in me and pushing me to reach higher. But even then, I felt the weight of everything we were about to face. With me moving to Zurich in September 2019 changed everything. Deep down, I knew he wouldn't adapt in the way I needed him to.

It crushed me when he started making subtle comments about my weight, leaving workout exercise videos around the bedroom like I wouldn't notice. He has no idea how much pressure I'm under. I've been stress-eating just to cope, and I don't even have the energy to think about exercising. My job demands everything I have, and I never felt like he was there to support me. Instead of helping me find balance, he just focused on his own routine—working out, watching TV, and taking long lunch breaks—while I struggled to keep everything together.

The move to Zurich was a turning point. It could have brought us closer, but instead, it pushed us further apart. His accusations that I'm controlling or neglectful hit hard. I'm doing everything I can to keep us afloat, and there's no room left for me to meet his emotional needs or spend hours watching TV with him. I barely sleep as it is, and I've realised how little I do for myself anymore. Despite everything, I'm grateful for the good times we've had. Almost 20 years of marriage is no small thing. We've had moments of real joy—family vacations, celebrations with friends, and quiet, ordinary days that felt special. He's taught me so much, and I'll always be thankful for that. But as I reflect, I see how those happy times have faded. The connection we once had is gone, and I've come to accept that this is the end. This isn't about a lack of love or respect; it's about reclaiming who I am and protecting my children from further pain.

It's hard to face the truth. To the outside world, he still seems perfect. But underneath, there's a disconnect that I can't ignore anymore. My old childhood pattern of making myself small and shrinking back and not really expressing my true feelings to keep the peace came at the greatest cost – my marriage. I've replayed so many moments in my mind, wondering if I could have done more or spoken up sooner. I regret not being more assertive, but even when I tried, it felt like he wasn't listening. His recent actions have made it even clearer how far apart we are. It's painful to realise how easily he puts his own needs first while mine have been ignored for so long. I feel like I've been pretending to be the perfect wife, managing everything while neglecting myself. I can't keep living this way.

To the outside world, we may still look like a perfect couple, but that's just a facade. As Elizabeth Gilbert said, "To be fully seen by somebody, then, and be loved anyhow—this is a human offering that can border on miraculous." We've reached a point where we can't go back. We have to find a way forward that works for both of us.

Our boys are older now, and they see more than I'd like to admit. It breaks my heart to know they've noticed the cracks in our relationship. They've no doubt lost some respect for their father because of his inconsistencies. I've tried to be steady for them, but it's been so hard.

Years ago, I didn't leave after I suspected him of infidelity because I was too scared. I feared the unknown and what it would mean for my boys. But that fear doesn't hold me anymore. I want us to grow as parents and build a healthy environment for our children, even if that means letting go of our marriage.

Looking ahead, I hope we can co-parent with honesty and put our children first. They need to know that we both love them, even if we're no longer together. This journey has been incredibly difficult, but I feel a sense of peace in my decision. I'm learning to honour my needs while thinking about what's best for my children. This isn't the end of love or gratitude for the man I married. It's the start of a new chapter where I can find myself again and create a better life for my children.

Implementing My Decision and Communicating with Our Children

By April 2021, after eight long and exhausting months of living together with Emmett, everything felt unbearable after the fateful day when it all fell apart. The home that had once been full of laughter and joy now felt empty and cold. It wasn't home anymore—it was just a place where we existed. We barely spoke, except when we had to talk about the boys, like their school schedules, meals, or chores. It was like we were living in separate worlds under the same roof. I found myself locking my bedroom door more and more, retreating into that small space just to feel some kind of escape. The boys began to notice. They'd ask me why I locked my bedroom door, their innocent faces full of curiosity. I didn't want to tell them the truth. I made up excuses about needing privacy because I couldn't bear to admit I was afraid. I didn't want them to know how tense and anxious I felt all the time. But kids are smart. Even if they didn't fully understand, I could see in their eyes that they felt something was wrong. The silence between Emmett and me was so heavy that it spoke louder than words, and the boys could sense it.

Finally, I made the decision to send Emmett a letter through my lawyer, asking for a divorce. I thought it would be a relief—a chance to breathe again, to reclaim my life. But instead of feeling free, I felt more trapped than ever. Emmett changed completely. He became angry and bitter, someone I barely recognised. The only time he spoke to me was to make unreasonable demands. By June 2021, he finally moved out—but only after I agreed to his demands. To make it worse, he refused to grant me a divorce despite my offering to share our marital assets equally. Instead, he agreed to a separation, which meant I'd have to wait two more years before I could truly move on. It felt like I was stuck, unable to move forward, no matter how hard I tried.

Telling the boys about the separation was one of the hardest things I've ever done. We sat them down at the dining table, and my heart felt like it was going to burst out of my chest. I could see the confusion and sadness on their faces as we explained. Their wide eyes said it all—they didn't understand why this was happening, and I knew their world was changing in ways they couldn't yet imagine. Watching their innocence fade broke my heart. I wanted to protect them from the pain, but I knew I had to be honest with them. And then, Emmett made it worse. Right there at the table, he told the boys that I was the one who wanted the divorce and that it is not what he wanted. My heart sank. I could see the confusion and anger on their faces as they tried to process his words. Suddenly, they were looking at me like I was the villain, the one responsible for breaking up our family. I could almost see them trying to figure out why I would do something so terrible.

After that conversation, the boys were hurt and upset. They looked at me differently—sad and maybe a little angry, too. They'd ask me, "Why did you want this, Mom?" Their voices were shaky, their little hearts breaking. I tried to explain, to tell them about the pain I'd been living with, but the words never seemed enough. I felt like I was drowning, trying to be strong for them while my own heart was shattering into pieces.

Truths Unveiled: Confronting the Dark Heart of Deception

Across the Chasm

In that moment, heavy hangs the air,

A heart once full, now tethered to despair.

Uncertainty looms like a shadowed night,

As anger battles compassion's gentle light.

How did love, once vibrant, fray at the seams?

Two souls now adrift in shattered dreams.

Opposite sides of a chasm they stand,

A gulf carved by choices, too vast to understand.

A web of deception, spun tight with intent,

His narcissistic grasp, a cruel testament.

She seeks the truth, but finds only pain,

In a labyrinth of lies, where trust is in vain.

Each word, a weapon, each silence, a scar,

As he rewrites their story, a distant, cruel star.

Her identity frays, her spirit besieged,

By the chaos he conjures, her peace, he's impeached.

The law, dressed in jargon, a cold, distant friend,

Fails to grasp nuances where hearts often bend.

Is justice a ledger, or can it be felt?

In the throes of this battle, her spirit is dealt.

Years slip like sand through an hourglass cracked,

Her strength wanes beneath the weight of his act.

Yet amidst the exhaustion, a flicker of light,

A realisation blooms in the depth of the night.

She cannot rewrite what's written in stone,

Nor change the man who has turned into bone.

But in her own hands, the power resides,

To shift from the struggle, to embrace her own tides.

Her children's futures, the legacy she'll weave,

A heritage rich, not a burden to grieve.

In their laughter, she finds her own song,

A melody of healing, where she can belong.

Forgiveness, not for him, but for her weary soul,

A gift she unwraps, a means to feel whole.

She reflects on the past, with compassion and grace,

Understanding the pain, yet reclaiming her space.

In sharing her story, her strength is unveiled,

Transforming her anguish, where once she had failed.

A testament woven from threads of her fight,

A narrative forged in resilience and light.

For true freedom whispers from deep within,

Where scars tell of battles, but never of sin.

As she steps into dawn, with lessons in tow,

She carries her truth, and the strength to let go.

So here stands a woman, reborn from the storm,

With grace as her armour, a heart now transformed.

Ready to face what the future may bring,

With courage and love, she'll rise and take wing.

In this chapter, I have used a different style to the broader book; I've written a fictitious story to show how even a small lie can grow and take over a person's life, leading a couple to question everything they thought they knew about love. The story is a powerful reminder of how dishonesty, no matter how small it seems at first, can have serious consequences over time.

This fictitious story is told from the woman's point of view to reflect the overall tone of this book. Her thoughts, feelings, and experiences shape the narrative, but it's important to remember that her perspective doesn't include the man's side of things. He probably sees what happened very differently and might have feelings or reasons that she doesn't fully understand. This difference shows how personal experiences can shape how we see relationships and the truth.

As the story unfolds, the woman looks back on her life—the happy moments, the challenges, and the way trust between them started to break down because of that one small lie. Each part of the story reveals how her idea of love and partnership has changed, forcing her to face tough questions about what's real and honest in their relationship.

The story reflects how complicated relationships can be and helps the reader understand how important it is to have empathy when dealing with different viewpoints. She also hopes for enough respect and kindness between her and the man to allow both of them to hold onto their own opinions without anger. By trying to understand each other's sides, she believes they can begin to heal and grow, even after facing betrayal.

In the end, this story isn't just about her journey. It encourages people to talk openly about honesty and the impact of their choices. The story is a reminder that love is powerful, but it's also delicate and needs truth and understanding to survive.

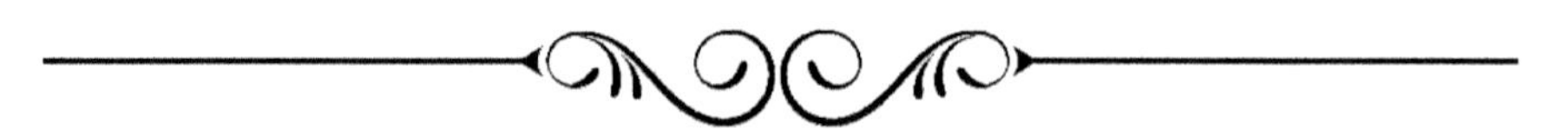

Shadows of Identity: A Journey Through Love, Deception, and Redemption

In early 90's, a young man arrived in South Africa, his heart full of dreams and hopes for a brighter future. He was excited to start at a well-known university, a place he believed would open doors to endless opportunities. But South Africa was going through a difficult time. Apartheid was ending, and the country was filled with tension and violence as people struggled for freedom and equality.

This young man came from Lesotho and had stepped into a township for "black" people, a lively but deeply scarred South African community. It was a place where joy and sadness mixed together. Children laughed and played in the streets, but the remains of oppression were everywhere. The smell of home-cooked meals filled the air, yet harsh rules still shaped life. The Group Areas Act dictated where people could live, crushing their dreams and limiting their freedom.

For this African man, the chance to start fresh was exciting but also terrifying. He felt both hope and fear. Eventually, he made a choice that would change his life forever. He got a South African document through unclear and questionable means. He didn't mean to hurt anyone, but this decision—possibly made out of desperation—created a tangle of lies and truths he would carry for years.

At first, he likely felt both thrilled and nervous as he held the identity book in his hands. It had his name and birth date, but it told a story that wasn't his. This document was his key to a better life, but it also hid his real identity—a secret that would follow him everywhere.

Year after year, he built a life in South Africa. He got a job, paid taxes, and married the woman he loved. On the surface, it seemed like he was living the dream. But deep down, he always feared someone would find out the truth. How could such a small lie grow into something that might ruin everything?

In 2000, everything came crashing down. After visiting his mother in Lesotho, he returned to South Africa, only to be stopped at the border. Officials took his passport due to an error on the document, and he suddenly felt the weight of his actions come down on him like a heavy storm. He wasn't just trying to get back to South Africa; he was trying to return to his wife, the woman he loved, who was waiting for him so they could start a new life together in Lisbon.

Detained in a cold, unwelcoming centre, the walls seemed to close in on him. Panic set in as he realised the seriousness of his situation. His voice shook as he called his wife, begging for her help. She rushed to him, her heart racing with fear and confusion. At that moment, she didn't know the full extent of his past. She only knew the man she loved was in trouble.

When she arrived, she was puzzled. He explained it as a mix-up, an administrative error. She believed him, partly because she had her own struggles with bureaucratic mistakes. Her birth certificate had caused her issues in the past, so she could relate. But while she saw it as a simple error, he knew it was something much bigger. This moment marked the first crack in their marriage—a secret he kept from her that would linger without her knowing.

With the help of an expert, they quickly made a plan. They travelled back to Lesotho together to sort out his papers. It was a stressful time, filled with long days and a lot of uncertainty. Through all the chaos, they clung to the hope of building a future together. Soon after, they set their sights on Lisbon, ready to start a new chapter in their lives. It seemed like they were leaving the past behind, but he couldn't shake the guilt and fear that came with his secret.

Over time, he realised just how delicate identity can be. It can be broken so easily but still hold so much power. In his wife's arms, he felt the strength of love—strong enough to rise above lies—but he also knew the truth would always be a part of their story. It was a reminder of how hard it is to balance hope and reality, and how much courage it takes to face the consequences of deception.

What stopped him from being honest with his wife at that moment? Why didn't he admit that there was a problem? If he had told her the truth, they might have worked together to fix the situation quickly and appropriately. Instead, he decided to shoulder the burden alone, a choice that would weigh him down for years. One lie had led to another, and now the web of deception was growing more complicated by the day. This single choice sowed seeds of doubt and led to the question of whether what they had was real love in his wife's heart.

As time went by, their life in Lisbon became busy and full. Their days were filled with the happy chaos of raising their children, the demands of work, and the joys of building a family. Still, every now and then, his wife would bring up the issue of the administrative error with the identity document.

"We really need to sort this out," she'd remind him, concern in her voice. He would nod, smiling reassuringly. "Don't worry," he'd say. "We'll handle it next time we're in South Africa. We'll get someone to help us do it properly." But every time, the promise faded into the background, forgotten amid the demands of everyday life.

Years went by, and the document stayed hidden, a ticking time bomb in their filing cabinet. In 2014, his wife decided to apply for South African citizenship for their children, who had been born in Lisbon. Confidently, she gathered all the necessary documents and went to the South African consulate. She thought it would be a straightforward process.

But then came an unexpected request. "We need your husband's South African ID to process the children's citizenship," the official said.

Her heart sank as she asked him later, "Where's your South African ID? I know they took your passport, but we need this for the children's citizenship application."

He hesitated, then replied, "I lost it years ago. Remember, we agreed to fix it next time we go to South Africa?"

Her frustration bubbled up. "We can't keep putting this off. I'll contact someone in South Africa who can help us sort it out."

A few weeks later, she got a response. The agency explained that only her husband could resolve the issue. He would have to go to the Home Affairs office in South Africa himself.

"Fine," he said, sounding resigned. "I'll deal with it when we go back, I promise."

But life moved on. Between caring for their children and managing busy jobs, the problem slipped further down their list of priorities.

Then came 2018, a year that changed everything. Their marriage, once full of love and shared dreams, was falling apart. Feeling trapped and unhappy, his wife decided to file for divorce. As she gathered paperwork for her lawyer, she stumbled upon something unexpected.

Digging through their filing cabinet, her fingers landed on a document she didn't recognise. Curious, she pulled it out. It was his South African identity document—the one he had claimed was lost.

At first, the document seemed unremarkable, but as she looked closer, unease crept in. Some inconsistencies needed to be clarified and raised questions. The administrative error became more apparent, it was much more significant than what she believed.

A few weeks later, during a tense meeting with their divorce attorneys, she confronted him, seeking clarity on the inconsistencies. He reacted defensively, shouting across the room. His lawyer quickly brushed off her concerns, saying it was irrelevant. But to her, it wasn't just about the accuracy of facts that affected legalities. It was about trust and inadvertently connecting someone else to your untruths. How could he dismiss something so important, something that flaws important legal documents in their joint lives but could unravel their life, which was built on trust and love together?

Due to the complete lack of acknowledgement of the issue, she was left with no choice but to seek legal advice in South Africa. The recommendation was clear: the only way to fix this mess was to remove his South African identity document from the population register, enabling other documents carrying the error to be corrected. Correcting this mistake was critical to enabling their children to be recognised as South Africans when applying for citizenship, but this solution relied entirely on his cooperation.

As she grappled with the situation, her emotions were a mix of anger, sadness, and compassion. How had their lives come to this? How had they drifted so far apart, caught in a web of half-truths?

This story shows how one bad decision, even if made with good intentions or out of sheer desperation, can spiral into a tangle of deception and pain. The wife, caught in the fallout of her husband's actions, struggled not just with legal consequences but with the emotional toll of his choices. Their reality became a reminder of how fragile trust can be—and how important it is to face the truth, no matter how difficult it may seem.

The woman felt that her husband's narcissistic tendencies show through in how he constantly tries to control the narrative to be consistent with what he believed was the truth. He is convinced that his wife is only motivated by money and not by a real desire to fix the accuracy of the legal documentation. His refusal to face the truth keeps the lies growing, creating a mess that his wife has to navigate emotionally. The story became more complex and grew as more half-truths piled onto the narrative; each new discovery led to more confusion and problems. This is a common pattern with narcissists—they create chaos and wear down their opponent, hoping they'll give up. With every new lie, the husband traps his wife further, making this not just a legal fight but a personal struggle for her sense of justice and identity.

The emotional toll on the wife is deep. She starts to see that the legal system, which should help, is not built to handle her search for the truth. Every time she tries to use the law, it becomes clear how it can be twisted, allowing her husband's lies to take hold. This adds to her feeling of being alone. The legal process, full of confusing rules and siloed strategies, pulls her further from the core of her battle—seeking fairness and truth.

As the conflict drags on for years, the wife becomes emotionally drained. Her husband's behaviour continued to chip away at the confidence that she had been fighting so hard to reclaim. She begins doubting herself and even questioning her own experiences. She feels helpless, knowing the truth is buried under her husband's refusal to face his faults. This exhaustion marks a turning point for her. She realises the fight isn't just against him but also against a legal system that doesn't see the full picture of her struggle for truth and justice.

In a moment of clarity, the wife understands that she can't change her husband or the legal system. She can only change how she deals with them. This realisation gives her a sense of freedom. Instead of staying focused on the fight for the truth, she decides to focus on her own healing. Thinking about her children and their future, like their chance at South African citizenship, strengthens her resolve. She sees her heritage as a gift she can pass on to them, not as a burden tied to her past.

This shift in mindset helps her find a way to forgive—not for her husband's sake, but for her own peace. She looks back on their life together with a mix of sadness and understanding. She knows how much both her and her husband's actions to fix this error led to choices that hurt her and their family, but she also sees that holding onto that hurt will only keep her stuck. Letting go of the need for him or the legal system to validate her feelings becomes a key part of her healing.

Disclaimer: This story is a work of fiction.

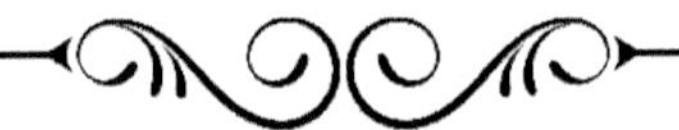

Conclusion

In sharing my journey, I find it helpful to reference a fictitious story that encapsulates my complex emotions. Reflecting on this narrative, I uncover profound parallels with my own life—particularly the way a single error can escalate into a significant turmoil, entangled in intricate legal disputes. More importantly, it compels me to confront deep-seated questions about the very foundations of love and trust in a relationship.

In the illustrative story, a woman wrestles with the painful reality of her partner's long-held secret, igniting doubts about the authenticity of their love. I, too, have felt the sharp sting of betrayal and deception, leading me to question the genuineness of Emmett affection for me. Through this process, I've come to realise that my quest for truth and justice, juxtaposed with his instinct for self-preservation, are fundamentally human responses. There is no blame to assign here—only an acceptance of our distinct journeys.

What began as a seemingly trivial administrative error ensnared the women in the story, morphing into something far more significant. This misstep reflected the trust they once shared, illuminating how a minor untruth can spiral into a tangled web of lies and deception.

Drawing from this story's lessons and personal experience, I unearthed a strength within myself that I hadn't known existed. I learned that letting go is not merely an act of liberation; it is essential for healing. By transforming my pain into a narrative of empowerment, I embarked on a journey towards moving forward. Accepting my truth and being honest about my experiences freed me from the shackles of the lies that once held me captive.

As highlighted in the story, there comes a moment when one must ask: Do truth and justice truly serve us when the pain and anxiety of legal battles are not only costly but also threaten to impact our children? Embracing acceptance is not a sign of weakness; rather, it is a recognition that the cost of the fight can hinder us from living a beautiful life. Just like the women in this story, I find solace in the knowledge that my heart knows the truth. Despite the challenges posed by a system that complicates the pursuit of justice, I choose to conserve my energy, comforted by the fact that I have done my utmost to live authentically. The truth matters more to me than anything else, and now it is time to let go.

In sharing my story, I take a powerful step towards self-acceptance, reminding myself of the immense courage required to embrace the future, even when the past has left its scars. Ultimately, this narrative transcends the impact of my husband's actions, just as the woman in the story conveys; it is about reclaiming my power, discovering my path to healing, and recognising that true freedom originates from within. As I look ahead, I carry with me the lessons I've learned and the resilience I've built, prepared to face whatever lies ahead with an open heart and renewed courage.

As Maya Angelou wisely noted, "I can be changed by what happens to me. But I refuse to be reduced by it." This sentiment echoes in my heart as I forge a new path, resolute in my commitment to living authentically and embracing the future with hope.

From Corporate Shadows to Clarity: Breaking Free

In the shadows of apartheid's cruel embrace,

A girl with dreams like distant, starlit grace,

Born into a family of eleven, she learned to fight,

Yet beneath the surface, scars whispered at night.

Emotional wounds from a land torn apart,

A young soul yearning, driven by her heart,

In a cacophony of voices, her own fell silent,

Fuelled by a fire to excel, to be defiant.

Eight years in the South African corporate grind,

Where she donned a mask, her true self confined,

Fearful of rejection, of never belonging,

Each day a battle, her spirit slowly thronging.

Then London beckoned with promises bright,

But amidst the chaos, her heart lost its light,

Her marriage frayed, twins clinging to her side,

She drifted further from the joy she once eyed.

Switzerland's beauty, a façade for her pain,

The relentless demands left her feeling insane,

At the edge of despair, exhausted and hollow,

She paused to reflect, daring to follow.

For eleven long months, she sought her own truth,

To reclaim her voice, to resurrect her youth,

Awakening to the truth that success dressed in gold,

Was but a mirage, a tale often told.

No longer shackled by corporate chains so tight,

She discovered her essence, her inner light,

Choosing only that which ignites her soul,

Focusing on passions that make her whole.

Executive titles may fade like the dusk,

But her happiness blooms, free from the husk,

With ego's games left far in the past,

She embraces a life that's authentic and vast.

So let her journey ignite a spark in us all,

To heed the whispers of our hearts' fervent call,

For in the depths of struggle and strife,

We can rise, like her, to a radiant life.

Navigating Identity and Career Growth in the South Africa's Landscape

Reflecting on my career journey in South Africa, I am enveloped in a blend of emotions—acceptance, gratitude, and a profound appreciation for the experiences that have shaped my path. As a young woman, I was driven by a determined but naive ambition to become a lawyer, convinced that the legal profession was my destiny. However, the reality of university life quickly dismantled that vision. The sight of towering textbooks seemed to mock me, and the relentless pressure to excel became a source of constant distress. What I once viewed as my life's calling turned into a burden of shame, as I wrestled with the high expectations I had placed upon myself.

The hours spent in the library became battles against a language that felt foreign and unyielding, leaving me lost and inadequate. Yet, within that despair came a crucial turning point: I accepted my struggle. This acknowledgement marked the beginning of a new chapter. I let go of the rigid confines of law and embraced the more relatable field of Social Science. Born from vulnerability, this decision set me on an unexpected path that led to the corporate world. Sometimes, life's most profound shifts stem from moments of uncertainty.

One memory stands out vividly—the day Charles, a manager at the store where I worked to fund my studies, saw potential in me that I hadn't yet recognised. It was a quiet but transformative moment, as if the universe had conspired to bring us together. His belief reignited a spark within me, long extinguished by self-doubt. With a mix of excitement and apprehension, I accepted his invitation to join the Retail Management Trainee program at a prominent retail organisation in 1994. This serendipitous turn of events marked the beginning of a journey filled with challenges and immense growth.

In 1999, I took another leap of faith by joining a leading FMCG multinational, a move that would change my career trajectory. Kim, the HR Director who hired me despite my lack of HR experience, saw potential that I hadn't yet realised. Her confidence in me opened doors to opportunities I hadn't imagined. It felt like another serendipitous alignment in my journey, nudging me toward a calling in Human Resources. This space became both a test of my abilities and an expansion of my worldview, revealing paths I never thought to explore. Each career twist seemed guided by an invisible force, leading me to opportunities that were both daunting and rewarding.

Reflecting on these formative experiences, I am grateful for how they shaped my understanding of leadership and community. Growing up in apartheid South Africa, I carried deep emotional childhood wounds that profoundly influenced my identity. Being labelled "coloured" marked me as different in a divided society, amplifying my sense of isolation amid systemic discrimination. I often felt caught between two worlds, grappling with a quest for belonging in an environment fraught with rejection.

At home, my parents' struggles created an emotional distance that added to my feelings of abandonment. Their grief over the loss of my older brother cast a long shadow over our family, leading to an uneven distribution of love and attention among the ten remaining children. As a child, I learned to navigate a chaotic landscape of emotional neglect, yearning for connection that always felt elusive. Books became my refuge, transporting me to worlds where I could escape the weight of my reality.

The societal expectations placed upon me intensified these burdens. Growing up amidst challenges like alcoholism and drug abuse, I felt a constant pressure to rise above my circumstances while struggling with my own insecurities. The tension between the expectation to succeed and my self-doubt left lasting emotional scars. Even in my corporate journey, I questioned my place in environments that often felt alien.

The early days of my corporate career in the 1990s shaped my resilience but also distanced me from my true self. Navigating a corporate culture that prioritised survival over authenticity required me to wear masks and adapt to unspoken rules. Each day felt like a performance, as I feared exposing any vulnerability.

Over time, I constructed a persona that strayed far from my essence. In my innocence, I absorbed life's experiences without the tools to process them. Trivial moments morphed into invisible chains, binding me to a narrative I hadn't chosen. These unspoken wounds became a defining part of me, until I realised that confronting them was the key to liberation. Now, as I look back, I find an ironic beauty in my journey: I achieved success in a world that often felt distant from my authentic self. By embracing my past, I've unlocked a future filled with possibility. Guided by gratitude for the lessons learned and resilience forged through adversity, I carry a deeper understanding of myself and the world. This understanding is now my source of pride.

Navigating Identity and Career Growth in London and Switzerland

As I reflect on the past two decades of my career across Europe, I am overwhelmed by a deep sense of gratitude. My journey has been nothing short of extraordinary—a rich tapestry of experiences that have shaped both my leadership and the organisations I've had the privilege to serve.

When I first arrived in Europe, the path ahead was a mix of uncertainty and promise. I vividly recall those initial days in HR at a leading FMCG multinational. Those moments were filled with learning opportunities that laid the foundation of my career. It was here that I first bridged the gap between talent strategies and business objectives, uncovering the transformative potential of strategic HR. With sleeves rolled up, I immersed myself in designing professional learning initiatives, aligning talent development with the company's overarching goals.

As the years passed, I found myself leading HR teams across multinational companies, navigating the complexities of cross-cultural environments. The challenge was both daunting and invigorating. I facilitated dialogues among diverse teams, fostering collaboration and trust. My leadership style resonated with colleagues, empowering us to tackle challenges and emerge stronger. Witnessing high-performance teams evolve was among the most rewarding aspects of my journey. I also encountered transformative milestones—mergers, acquisitions, joint ventures, and divestitures. I recall the adrenaline of managing a complex acquisition, striving to integrate contrasting corporate cultures. These moments tested my patience and strategic insight, positioning me as a driver of change and synergy.

My commitment to digital transformation has remained unwavering. One of my proudest achievements involved leading an analysis of HR operations across multiple countries. This initiative not only unveiled operational complexities but also ushered in a data-driven culture that revolutionised processes and enhanced the employee experience. The resulting surge in efficiency and cost savings was immensely fulfilling.

Over the years, I've had the privilege of working with remarkable people. Collaborating with executive leadership teams and engaging with the C-suite for 16 of my 20 years in Europe has shaped my understanding of leadership. True leadership, I've learned, is rooted in trust and empowerment. Above all, I treasure helping individuals unlock their potential. Watching others realise their capabilities has been a source of immense pride and fulfilment. Whether through conversations, workshops, or tailored development plans, guiding people toward their goals has been a privilege.

To deepen my ability to support others, I pursued a coaching qualification, which honed my skills in facilitating meaningful growth. As the book *Co-Active Coaching* reminds us, "The client is the expert in their own life." This philosophy underpins my approach, empowering individuals to take ownership of their journeys while I guide and support their development. My passion for helping others make the most of their strengths goes beyond just a career goal. It's at the heart of how I approach leadership. I'm committed to creating an environment where people feel valued, supported, and inspired to reach their full potential. Personal and professional growth is a shared journey, and I feel lucky to be part of it. Every success story lights a fire in me and reminds me of the powerful impact we can have on each other when we focus on growth and development.

I am profoundly grateful to the remarkable leaders who have believed in me and championed my development throughout my career. While many individuals have contributed to my journey, a select few have left an indelible mark, each imparting invaluable lessons: **Paul, Rebecca, Richard, Matsui San, and Padma**.

Paul recognised my potential and facilitated my secondment to the company headquarters in London. His unwavering faith in me fundamentally transformed my trajectory, teaching me the vital importance of recognising potential in others. Moving to London marked a pivotal turning point in my life, allowing me to be valued for who I am rather than the colour of my skin—a stark reminder of my upbringing in South Africa during apartheid.

Rebecca believed in my capabilities to establish a professional Academy for HR and ardently supported my pursuit of a Master's in International HR Management at Cranfield School of Management. She exemplified the power of encouragement and the profound impact of investing in someone's growth. This program not only deepened my passion for HR but also equipped me with a richer understanding of the profession, propelling my career to new heights.

Richard, through his exemplary leadership, demonstrated how to navigate difficult decisions with integrity. His trust in me instilled courage and reinforced my commitment to my values, reminding me that true leadership is characterised by compassion and the strength to remain resolute even in challenging times. Collaborating with leaders like Richard during tough decisions fortified my resolve to uphold my principles.

Matsui San shared his wisdom and illuminated the intricacies of Japanese culture, broadening my understanding of diversity and emphasising the importance of humility as a leader. Achieving what once seemed impossible was not easy, but Matsui San's unwavering commitment motivated me to strive for excellence without compromising my integrity.

As evident from our first meeting, **Padma's** steadfast belief in my capabilities inspired me to embrace new challenges. Her trust in me—having hired me not once but twice—taught me that compassion and support can empower individuals to realise their full potential. Padma was also instrumental in my relocation to Switzerland, a transformative experience that brought me calm and clarity in my life.

These leaders offered unique advice and guidance, mentoring me and fostering a sense of belonging, even when the corporate world felt daunting. They supported me not out of obligation but because they genuinely cared about my success. Their encouragement has given me the confidence and determination to push boundaries and explore new opportunities. I am deeply thankful for their profound impact on my life and career.

Looking back on my time working in global multinational companies across Europe, I see how those experiences shaped me. It was an exciting mix of growth and learning that opened my heart and mind. Traveling to new and different places wasn't just part of the job; it was a chance to experience other cultures and perspectives. Each destination became a new chapter in my story, filled with lessons that deepened my understanding of people and the world.

Rediscovering Authenticity: A Journey from Corporate Success to Personal Fulfillment

To many, my life might seem glamorous and full of adventure. While that's partly true, what really enriched my life were the meaningful experiences. I poured my heart into my work, driven by a passion that often consumed me. Sometimes, I became too attached to the title and prestige of my roles—they seemed to define who I was. My title felt like a badge of honour, showing the hard work I had put in. But beneath the shiny surface of what looked like a dream life, I found a deeper truth. My journey hasn't just been about achievements or the excitement of new experiences. It has been about transformation—learning resilience and discovering the power of empathy. Each opportunity wasn't just a career milestone; it was a chance to face challenges and embrace change. With every setback, I found strengths I didn't know I had. And with every victory, I learned to value humility and gratitude.

Because of my mentors and experiences, I've realised that real fulfilment doesn't come from titles or roles. It comes from the connections we make and the positive impact we have on others. I carry with me the lessons from leaders who believed in me, the memories of places I've visited, and the incredible people I've met. My journey has become a story of growth, woven together with support, learning, and a constant effort to be my best self. But I still wonder if I'm truly that best version of myself. As my life became more polished, I started feeling empty inside, like something important was missing.

The shadows of my early corporate days in the mid-1990s linger and weigh heavily on me. They remind me of the walls I built around myself—walls that now feel like chains, keeping me stuck in a version of myself that doesn't feel real. I feel disconnected, like I'm trapped between who I've become and the vibrant person I used to be. That bright, energetic spirit has dimmed, leaving behind a shell of who I once was. I've created a façade to survive in a world that often values blending in over being genuine.

In trying so hard to fit into the corporate world, I lost parts of myself. I became someone who performed instead of someone who lived authentically. Each day felt like acting in a play, putting on masks to hide my vulnerabilities. I got really good at hiding my self-doubt and the constant need for approval that churned inside me. As Brené Brown says, "We can't practice compassion with other people if we can't treat ourselves kindly." To my colleagues, I looked like a confident leader, speaking my mind with authority. But inside, I was scared. I carefully avoided topics that might make me look foolish or shake up the system too much. I learned to follow the unspoken corporate rules, suppressing my emotions and staying guarded. It reminded me of my early career days in South Africa, where I felt I couldn't show weakness. I feared being judged, scrutinised, or rejected.

Over time, I started to dislike the person I was becoming. I felt less and less like myself. When I faced situations that didn't feel right—whether a toxic workplace or a conflict with my values—I would leave gracefully. While some career moves were for better opportunities, two key decisions were about refusing to tolerate unethical or toxic environments. As Adam Grant says, "Toxic workplaces can lead to a profound sense of isolation and frustration, where the very air feels heavy with distrust and competition." In senior roles, I saw the darker side of corporate life. Egos ruled, and backstabbing was common in the name of survival. Teamwork gave way to competition, and trust was hard to find.

More and more, I became frustrated with the gap between what some leaders claimed to stand for and how they actually behaved. This disconnect left me feeling disillusioned. As an HR leader, I was the go-to person for colleagues who needed to vent about their struggles. They often shared their disappointment about the difference between the company's values and their everyday reality. Fear of retaliation kept most from speaking out or demanding change. Carrying these secrets became a heavy burden. A job I once loved started to feel like a weight I couldn't escape.

At times even my peers became part of the competitive game, each one striving to outshine the rest for the next promotion. The teamwork I once enjoyed turned into a contest, leaving me feeling isolated. Interactions became calculated, every move deliberate. I learned to question motives behind compliments and offers to help. The corporate camaraderie I had once cherished had turned into something I no longer recognised.

Now, I yearn to feel connected to my true self again, to let go of the constant performance and be genuine. I think back to a time when I could laugh freely and share my thoughts without fear. When my ideas came naturally, unfiltered and full of enthusiasm. But over time, I got tangled in expectations—those of my colleagues, my bosses, and even myself. I became an actor, wearing a mask that hid the real me. That spark I once had has dimmed, replaced by the exhausting need to perform and fit into a mould that feels far too tight.

This inner conflict was mixed with a deep sense of loss—not just of who I used to be but of all the chances I missed while trying so hard to fit in. I grieve the moments when I stayed silent instead of speaking up, letting fear control my decisions and silence my voice. These regrets weigh on me, constantly reminding me of how much of my true self I gave up just to conform. Now, the person I am feels far away, like a faint echo drowned out by the constant noise of surviving in the corporate world. I can't help but question my place in life and even who I really am.

With the breathtaking backdrop of Switzerland's majestic mountains and serene lakes, their beauty enveloping me like a comforting embrace, I increasingly questioned: Who am I, really? In those quiet moments of reflection, I began to see that my daily life often felt like acting in a play. It felt like the real me was hidden behind the roles I had to play. Was I truly being myself when my heart and mind seemed to be pulling in completely different directions? This conflict felt like a heavy knot of anxiety inside me, tightening every day. In Michael Singer's book *The Untethered Soul*, he describes this kind of turmoil as more than just a problem—it's a wake-up call to explore deeper parts of who we are. I realised I had to make a change. I needed to quiet my overthinking mind and let my real self take the lead. By letting go of all the mental noise, I hoped to break down the barriers holding me back from living fully, allowing my heart to guide me and my spirit to feel free again.

Feeling completely burnt out from long hours and an endless schedule, I was caught in a storm of emotional chaos. I knew I wasn't alone in this—everyone around me seemed silently exhausted too.

Years of insomnia had drained me, leaving me a shell of who I used to be. On top of that, I was going through the painful process of separating from my husband, with the collapse of my marriage constantly looming over me. My teenage sons needed me more than ever, but I felt like I was barely holding myself together. I tried to be there for them, but I was struggling with feelings of failure. Therapy sessions became a lifeline for me, helping me stay connected to who I used to be. Even so, each session felt like a battle against the overwhelming sadness.

And then there was my body. I hardly recognised the person in the mirror anymore. Poor eating habits and neglect had taken their toll, and I realised my health was another victim of the corporate grind. I knew I needed to make a change. If I didn't, I feared losing not just my identity but everything that made me whole.

I remember the moment I decided to step away from corporate life. It was terrifying but necessary. I felt like I was standing on the edge of a cliff, ready to leap into the unknown. My heart was pounding with fear and excitement at the same time. But deep down, I knew it was the right decision. I needed time to reflect and figure out who I really was. As soon as I made the choice, it felt like a weight was lifting off my shoulders, even just a little.

That decision marked a turning point for me—a chance to reconnect with myself and figure out what I truly wanted from life. I took an 11-month break from the corporate world, and those months turned into a journey of self-discovery and healing.

As the months passed, the fast pace of corporate life faded away, leaving behind a quiet stillness. In that stillness, I began to feel hope again, like the first rays of sunlight after a long, dark night. I started writing again, pouring my thoughts onto paper. Writing became a way to sort through my emotions and find clarity. Each word I wrote felt like a step closer to finding myself. The steady rhythm of my pen was like a lifeline, helping me rediscover my voice.

I also started spending more time in the breathtaking Swiss landscape, immersing myself in nature like never before. I wandered through lush green valleys and along sparkling lakes, breathing in the crisp, fresh air that filled my lungs with a sense of renewal. The rustling leaves of the towering trees and the melodious songs of birds flitting through the branches reminded me that beauty and vitality still thrived, both in the world around me and within my own spirit. The majestic mountains stood as silent guardians, their grandeur instilling a deep sense of calmness that enveloped me. Nature's delicate balance illustrated the cycles of life, revealing to me that, just like the changing seasons, I too could grow and heal in this serene embrace.

One of the most meaningful changes during this time was reconnecting with my role as a mother. For the first time in years, I was fully present with my kids. I took on the school drop-offs and pick-ups myself, and those 20-minute car rides became special moments filled with laughter and real connection. I embraced the messy, chaotic world of raising teenagers, realising how much I'd missed while they were growing up. Those everyday routines turned into precious opportunities to bond and rebuild our relationships.

I also started using my professional coaching skills to help others, offering pro bono sessions. I worked with people struggling to navigate the corporate world, helping them deal with office politics and avoid losing themselves in the process. Supporting others gave me a deep sense of purpose, and seeing their progress reminded me of the resilience we all have inside us.

I began to take better care of my body, giving it the attention it deserved. Slowly, it started to respond, almost as if it recognised my efforts to heal. I learned to meditate, finding peace in moments of silence. I also participated in ancient spiritual healing ceremonies, which helped me connect with traditions that resonated deeply with me. These experiences grounded me and gave me a stronger sense of connection to myself and the world around me.

During this journey, I discovered what I truly wanted from my career. It wasn't about big titles or status anymore. I wanted meaningful work that made a difference, without the toxic politics that often come with executive roles. I accepted that corporate dynamics wouldn't change, no matter where I worked. What I could control, however, was how I approached my life and work.

Looking back, I came to appreciate the lessons I learned during my corporate career. Each challenge, success, and failure shaped me and helped me grow. Late-night meetings and tough leadership decisions taught me about teamwork, leadership, and human connection. Every experience was a stepping stone toward greater self-awareness.

For most of us, having a job is a necessity, but I learned that it's possible to build resilience and stay true to yourself, even in challenging environments. I committed to protecting my well-being and maintaining my boundaries. This inner strength became my guide, helping me navigate the pressures of both work and personal life.

After 11 months, I decided to return to the corporate world, but this time in a smaller role. I wanted to see if I could bring everything I had learned into this new chapter. To my surprise, I found that I was much stronger and clearer about who I was and what I stood for. I allowed myself to be vulnerable and authentic, trusting that I could meet my responsibilities without getting caught up in office politics. I also learned to be compassionate, recognising that many people around me were struggling with their own fears and challenges.

The past 18 months in my most recent corporate role have been both demanding and rewarding. I've proven to myself that I can balance corporate life with my personal passions. I've continued coaching, finding joy in helping others discover their potential. Being part of a philanthropic foundation has also become a key part of my life. Working alongside people who share my commitment to protecting the planet and preserving ancient wisdom has given me a deeper sense of purpose. Together, we've listened to the stories of elders and environmental stewards, learning from their wisdom and working to build a sustainable future. These experiences have inspired me and reminded me of the importance of honouring the past while shaping a better tomorrow.

Through this journey, I've come to realise that corporate jobs, while necessary for financial stability, don't define who we are. They're a means to an end, often influenced by factors beyond our control. I've learned not to fear the unknown but to embrace it instead. Every day brings new opportunities, and change has the power to help us grow. My time in the corporate world has been an important chapter in my life. It taught me resilience, adaptability, and the importance of staying true to myself. Without these experiences, I wouldn't have discovered my true identity.

I'm grateful for all the opportunities my corporate career gave me. Working with executive teams was more than just a job. Many colleagues became mentors, teaching me valuable skills like negotiation, strategy, and diplomacy. In high-stakes meetings, I learned how to handle complex situations, understanding that clear communication is often the key to success. I found a balance between being assertive and empathetic and discovered that true leadership inspires and brings people together toward shared goals.

But as much as I gained, I also realised that climbing the corporate ladder wasn't for me. Chasing titles and promotions started to feel empty, like running after something that didn't truly matter. While each step up seemed like progress, it often came at the cost of my authentic self. The late nights, constant meetings, and endless demands drained my energy and spirit. In those quiet moments of reflection, I understood that true fulfilment doesn't come from titles or recognition—it comes from work that aligns with who I am and what I value most.

Now, I'm focused on projects that feed my soul. This change has been freeing. I've sought out work that challenges me intellectually and lets me contribute to meaningful causes. Coaching others has brought me immense joy, as I share the lessons I've learned to help others thrive. These connections and moments of growth feel deeply rewarding, reminding me that success isn't about individual achievements but about being part of something bigger.

For me, success now means choosing work that reflects my values—work that supports sustainability, social equity, and the preservation of ancient wisdom. It's about advocating for practices that benefit both people and the planet. Every decision I make is guided by a desire to stay true to my beliefs, not just climb the next rung of the ladder.

This new chapter is about creating a legacy that aligns with my core values. I want to build spaces where creativity and innovation can thrive and where people feel safe to explore their passions. I'm committed to supporting initiatives that protect the planet and honour ancient traditions, weaving these principles into modern solutions. This isn't just a career shift; it's a calling—a commitment to live in a way that reflects my beliefs.

I know this path won't always be easy. There will be challenges and moments of doubt. But I feel stronger knowing I'm staying true to myself. The corporate world will always be part of my story, but it no longer defines it. I'm writing my own narrative now, one rooted in authenticity, purpose, and a deep connection to life's bigger picture. Every step I take is intentional, reflecting my values and my belief that success is measured by the positive impact we have on others.

Standing on the edge of this new chapter, I feel a mix of excitement and nervousness. The future is uncharted, full of possibilities. I imagine expanding my coaching work beyond traditional boundaries—maybe into community workshops or wellness retreats that blend ancient practices with modern approaches. I dream of creating spaces where people can connect with themselves and with nature, finding belonging in a world that often feels disconnected.

Of course, fears creep in—the worry about financial stability or leaving behind the security of a familiar path. But I remind myself that growth requires taking risks. Life is always changing, and I've chosen to trust in that process.

Ultimately, this journey is about more than just my personal growth. It's about contributing to something greater. The lessons I've learned from corporate life, the people I've coached, and the wisdom shared by those preserving ancient knowledge have all shaped me. Together, they form a story of resilience, hope, and the belief that we can live authentically while making a difference in the world.

As I close this chapter and step into the next, I carry with me the lessons of my past and the dreams that propel me forward. The road ahead may be uncertain, but I move forward with confidence, ready to weave my story into the larger fabric of life, guided by passion, purpose, and the timeless wisdom of those who came before me.

In this spirit, I invite you to reflect on your own journey and the choices that define you. As I embrace this new chapter, I encourage you to seek paths that resonate with your true self, even in the face of uncertainty. Each step you take is an opportunity to align your actions with your values, foster meaningful connections, and create a legacy that truly reflects who you are. Together, let us move forward, courageous in our pursuit of authenticity and committed to making a meaningful impact in the world. Your story is waiting to be written—embrace it with open arms and a hopeful heart.

The Complexity of Love: From Attachment to Acceptance

The Paradox of Love

In the garden where emotions grow,

Love blooms bright but casts dark shadows,

A tender rose with thorns concealed,

Its beauty known, yet pain revealed.

It whispers sweetly in the night,

Yet stirs the heart to jealous fright,

A force that binds, a grip so tight,

In obsession's dance, it dims the light.

For love can twist, a serpent's coil,

In fear of loss, our hearts embroil,

With greed it taints, with wrath it stings,

A hollow echo of what true love brings.

Yet, in the silence of the soul,

A deeper love can make us whole,

When freed from chains of need and doubt,

It nurtures peace, it brings about.

Compassion flows like gentle streams,

In self-acceptance, we find our dreams,

With empathy, our spirits soar,

In love's true form, we're rich, not poor.

So here we stand, at love's great gate,

With choices vast, we shape our fate,

It holds the pain, it holds the grace,

A paradox that time can't erase.

For love can tear, and love can mend,

A bitter foe, a faithful friend,

In every heart, its song is sung,

The battle fierce, yet love is young.

Choose wisely then, as love unfolds,

In open hands, let go of holds,

For in this dance, both dark and light,

We find our truth, our inner sight.

Love has always been a puzzle for me—a mix of beauty and struggle that has shaped who I am. It's amazing and heartbreaking how love can drive us to do both wonderful and harmful things. On one hand, it can lead us to hurt ourselves and others. On the other, it's the gentle force that feeds our souls, helping us find peace and self-worth. This balance—the good and the bad—has been a big part of my life, teaching me that love can both lift us up and bring us down.

I remember the pain of love turning into obsession. The fear of losing someone would eat away at me, constantly whispering doubts in my mind. Jealousy would take over, making me act in ways I didn't like—greedy, controlling, and manipulative. What should have been something beautiful became heavy and overwhelming. I held onto love so tightly that it pushed me into dark places where my insecurity pretended to be love. During those times, I felt lost, stuck in a cycle of hurting myself and others because of my own fears.

But even in those tough moments, I found the other side of love—the kind that heals and grows. When I began to love with no strings attached, without fear or expectations, I felt myself change. The love I gave to myself and others, rooted in kindness and understanding, brought me a peace I had been longing for. It became my safe place, a way to care for my inner self. I realised that when love isn't tied to fear or need, it can guide me in the right direction.

This journey showed me the two sides of love. Its darker side brought out my worst traits, but its pure side gave me the chance to be my best self. How I approached love made all the difference. When I came to it with fear or desperation, it turned toxic and drained me. But when I leaned into love with respect and acceptance, it became a source of balance and purpose in my life.

Looking back, I see how my choices in love have shaped my life. After nearly 20 years of marriage and the incredible experience of raising my twin boys, I've come to a life-changing truth: learning to love myself is the key to everything. Until I truly loved myself, I couldn't fully give or receive the love I needed from others.

Still, even with all I've achieved, there were times when I felt empty and bitter. Despite the blessings in my life, something felt missing. That feeling led me on a journey of self-discovery and deeper love. Along the way, I've learned that real love starts with how we treat ourselves. It's a gift we give to ourselves first, which then spreads to others. When we embrace it fully, love has the power to light up even the darkest parts of our hearts.

In the following pages, I want to share my love story. It begins with my husband, whose presence brightened my life, and continues with my children, who brought a level of joy I never thought possible. Each relationship has been full of lessons, challenges, and moments of pure happiness. I'll also talk about how my relationships with family and friends have shaped my understanding of love, adding their own unique pieces to the puzzle. Finally, I'll explore how I learned to take care of myself, including how focusing on nutrition became an important way for me to practice self-love and nurture both my body and spirit.

Every story I share will show the two sides of love—the way it can lift us up and challenge us at the same time. Through these experiences, I've learned what it means to truly connect with others. I've gone from holding onto love out of fear to embracing it as a source of strength. This journey has helped me let go of my anxieties and become the love I was always meant to be.

Sarah Prout sums this up beautifully in her book *Be the Love* when she says, "When you learn to love yourself, you unlock the door to the greatest love of all—the love that flows effortlessly, freely, and abundantly." Her words deeply resonate with me because they reflect my own journey. By learning to care for myself, I've found the ability to love and be loved in a way that feels genuine and free.

I invite you to join me as I dive into this journey of love. Together, we'll explore the joy and sorrow, the lessons learned, and the way love can change us. Through these stories, I hope to show how embracing both the light and dark sides of love has led me to a fuller, more meaningful life. It's a path that has allowed me to stand not just as someone who loves but as someone who embodies love itself.

Love as a Partner: Embracing the Journey of Marriage

In recent years, as I started looking inward and trying to understand myself better, one question kept haunting me: What is love? It wasn't something I could ignore—it would pop into my head at the strangest times, like a shadow I couldn't escape. Did Emmett ever truly love me? Did I love him? What does love even mean? These questions swirled around, leaving me wondering if my family and I really knew how to give and receive love. Did I love my kids, or was it just a deep sense of responsibility? And the hardest question of all—did I even know how to love myself? These thoughts twisted and turned in my mind, becoming louder and more confusing. It felt like a storm in my head, drowning out any chance of finding real answers.

Eventually, I couldn't take it anymore. I had to break free from this endless cycle of doubt and confusion. Surely, with all the knowledge out there, someone must have figured out what love is. Feeling vulnerable, I decided to try something different—I asked my ChatGPT AI tool to write a poem about love. It wasn't a decision I made lightly, and I could almost imagine the judgment from others. Turning to an AI for answers about love might seem odd, even desperate. But I was desperate. I'm an introvert, someone who prefers the safety of my own thoughts, and I was still healing from the end of a 22-year relationship. I needed something, anything, to help me make sense of it all. Within seconds, the AI responded with a poem. I wasn't expecting much, but the words that appeared on my screen took my breath away. The poem was beautiful, with a depth and meaning that spoke to me in a way I hadn't expected. It felt like someone had reached into my heart and put my emotions into words.

That moment made me realise that answers can come from the most unexpected places. It wasn't just a poem; it was a small but powerful reminder that love—no matter how confusing or complex—has meaning if we're willing to look for it.

What is love?

Unconditional love, a boundless sea,

Where hearts roam wild and spirits free.

It knows no limits, no bounds, no end,

A timeless force, forever to defend.

In its embrace, flaws find solace sweet,

Imperfections cherished, hearts complete.

Through darkest nights and brightest days,

It guides, it comforts, in countless ways.

Unconditional love, a steady flame,

In joy and sorrow, it's still the same.

It doesn't fade with passing time,

But blooms eternal, sublime, divine.

It sees beyond the masks we wear,

To the essence of souls laid bare.

It's not possessive, nor does it control,

But honours autonomy, a sacred role.

It's not a transaction, tit for tat,

Nor does it falter at the drop of a hat.

It's not demanding, nor does it judge,

But nurtures growth with gentle nudge.

Unconditional love, a melody rare,

Whispered in the breeze, felt everywhere.

It's a gift we give, without expectation,

A timeless bond, a divine creation.

Tears rolled down my face, and I couldn't fully explain why. My body reacted before my mind could make sense of it all. A deep ache hit my stomach, almost like I was about to be sick. I realised that my body was trying to tell me something important. Those tears weren't just random; they were a release, a way to let go of sadness, loss, and grief.

As the days passed and turned into weeks, I started to reflect. Slowly, the heaviness I felt began to ease. I wasn't just grieving the end of a relationship—I was mourning a love I had never truly known. A poem I had read had stirred something in me, making me realise the kind of love I longed for but never had. I grieved for my younger self, for my 22-year relationship with Emmett, and for a marriage that didn't survive. It felt like I was mourning the version of myself that had never been fully loved or allowed to thrive.

Coming to terms with this truth wasn't easy. Part of me just wanted to bury the feelings, to distract myself and move on. But when I stopped to really think about it, I felt the weight of what love can mean—the good and the bad. I yearned for a love that felt complete, one that was unconditional and free. Yet, I realised I was still on this journey of understanding love—for myself and for others—and it wasn't something I could rush.

Looking back on my time with Emmett, I started to see the mix of love and loss that shaped our story. I remembered the early days when everything felt fresh and full of promise, though there was always a hint of sadness I couldn't quite put into words. One memory stood out: a trip to the Drakensberg mountains. It was supposed to be romantic and fun. I loved the wind in my hair as we rode horses and soaked in the beauty of nature. But even then, Emmett's words stung. "Why do you have to stare at every leaf on each tree we pass?" he asked, his tone mocking. At the time, I ignored it, desperate to feel loved and accepted. How often had I brushed off that same tone? I remembered how he talked about my background in Sydenham, as though it was something to be embarrassed about. Thinking back, I realised how often I had undervalued myself, blinded by my need for love and approval.

That moment in Drakensberg captured so much of what our relationship was like. Emmett was always pushing for the next big thing, the next adventure, the next success. He rarely stopped to appreciate what was right in front of us. At first, I thought he was encouraging me to aim higher, but soon, it felt like nothing I did was ever enough. We became the couple others admired from a distance, with financial success and a picture-perfect life. But behind closed doors, I felt a growing distance. His support turned into demands, and his kindness often felt like control. My worth seemed to depend on how well I could meet his endless expectations.

One memory still haunts me: during the construction of our holiday home in Benguela Cove, I saw a side of Emmett I couldn't ignore. He snapped at the construction workers, his voice filled with disdain, saying something that boiled down to, "I'm paying for this, so do as I say." It hit me like a slap. How many times had he spoken to me in that same way? In that moment, I saw him clearly—a man I no longer recognised, someone I wasn't sure I wanted to be with. The love that once felt warm now felt cold and distant, and I couldn't push that feeling away any longer.

Looking back, those small moments weren't small at all. They were signs of a relationship breaking down. On that Drakensberg trip, I just wanted to be happy, convinced love would be enough. But standing in our Benguela Cove home years later, surrounded by everything we had built, I felt the weight of all the beauty and pain we had shared. I started to realise that love shouldn't mean losing respect for yourself.

In 2021, I had another wake-up call. I went through a leadership review—a 360-degree feedback report from my colleagues. The results shocked me. Their view of me was so different from how I saw myself. It forced me to ask a hard question: Why didn’t I see my own value? After a lot of soul-searching, I understood that my low self-esteem came from the toxic patterns in my relationship with Emmett and unresolved pain from my past. His constant criticism and condescending words had worn me down, making me doubt myself. Ironically, on most occasions, his criticism was always wrapped in a sea of beautiful words, yet the essence of his message was jarring and painful. Even though we had good times, it became clear we were heading in different directions. The dreams we once shared were gone, leaving us both searching for something we couldn’t find in each other.

At one point, I got lost in a Netflix binge, watching one love story after another. It started with a poem I read on ChatGPT that stirred up a lot of emotions. Watching those shows and movies became my escape, a way to avoid facing reality—something I'd done since I was a kid. But when I finally came out of that binge, I reflected on what I had learned. The love stories I watched had a lot in common, and they taught me important lessons about love's many shapes and forms. I thought about the early days with Emmett when everything felt magical and new. It was like seeing the world in bright, vibrant colours. A single glance could light up my day, and our laughter felt like a secret treasure, something I believed would hold us together forever.

In those early years, I felt like I was living the dream. I was part of the popular crowd, going to parties, celebrating milestones, and enjoying the thrills of being young. Life seemed perfect, and our love felt unstoppable. When we moved to London in 2002 for my job, it was like stepping into the next chapter of our fairytale. My new job brought exciting travel opportunities, and for a while, it really felt like we were living a dream filled with endless possibilities. While my career was taking off, Emmett decided to take a break from his career and focus on earning a Master's Degree. He embraced the student life with excitement, throwing himself into his studies and the university environment. But while he was busy with this new chapter of his life, I often found myself alone on Friday nights, watching the lively city outside my window. He seemed to put everything ahead of me—his studies, his friends, and the nightlife. What once felt exciting now left me feeling lonely.

Instead of confronting these feelings, I pushed them down the way I'd learned to do as a child. I told myself it was my role as a wife to accept his absence, focus on the home, and not complain. When I finally tried to share my frustrations, it felt like talking to a brick wall. I remember one weekend when I opened up about feeling so alone while he was out enjoying himself. He shrugged it off, calling me insecure. That hurt deeply, and it felt like my feelings didn't matter. Over time, our relationship settled into a routine. The passion we once had turned into something distant, and the intimacy we shared felt more like an obligation than a real connection. It was in those years, before our children were born, that I first started to feel something wasn't right. The gap between us grew wider as time went on, and I didn't know then how much worse it would become after we had kids.

Everything changed when our twin boys were born in 2008. I'll never forget the joy of holding them for the first time. Emmett seemed excited to be a dad at first. In those early days, he was fully involved, playing with the boys and laughing with them. But as parenting got harder and we brought in a nanny to help, he slowly pulled back. He only seemed to show up when it was convenient for him. I wanted to share the joys and struggles of parenting with him—the sleepless nights, the endless diaper changes, the chaos of feeding twins—but he chose fun over responsibility. His excuse? "We have a nanny, so why should I do their work?"

I ended up doing everything—running the household, managing the kids, and trying to keep it all together. The twins needed constant attention, and even with a nanny, I was the one juggling schedules, planning meals, and making sure everything ran smoothly. I went back to work just three months after they were born, which added even more to my plate. Between work trips, preparing meals for Emmett, leaving instructions for the nanny, and handling all the household tasks, I was completely drained. Weekends were no better; they were filled with chores like cooking, shopping, and cleaning. I convinced myself that this was what love looked like—through acts of service and sacrifice. My upbringing had taught me to accept this as normal, but deep down, I felt like I was disappearing. I was exhausted and overwhelmed, but I kept going because I thought it was my duty as a wife and mother. It felt like I was stuck on a carousel, spinning faster and faster, with no way to get off.

In an effort to save our relationship, I introduced Emmett to Gary Chapman's book *The Five Love Languages.* I hoped it would help him understand what I needed—quality time and acts of service. But Emmett seemed to focus only on his own needs: physical touch and words of affirmation. Meanwhile, I was running on empty. I was barely sleeping, getting less than five hours a night, and over time I developed insomnia. Our intimate moments became just another task on the list. I felt used, as if my needs didn't matter at all. Resentment started building inside me, growing heavier with each passing day. At night, I would collapse into bed, feeling like our love was slowly unravelling. I wanted so badly for us to reconnect, to rediscover the magic we once had. But the more I tried to reach out, the further he seemed to drift away. I began to feel like I was fighting for our relationship all on my own.

Looking back at our photos, anyone would think I had nothing to complain about. We travelled the world, visiting incredible places like the beaches of Greece and the bustling streets of Morocco. Our lives looked perfect from the outside, full of family gatherings, birthdays, and holidays. But beneath that shiny surface, I often felt like a stranger in my own life. I spent so much time planning and preparing for these events—cooking, cleaning, hosting—that I felt more like a prop in the background than an active part of the story.

I once read about the idea of a "love tank," how love needs to be replenished to keep a relationship strong. Over the years, my love tank felt like it was leaking, slowly draining away. It was as if Emmett didn't see me as his partner anymore but as someone who existed to support his dreams. Even in our most private moments, I felt invisible. I started refusing his advances, and the frustration and anger that had been building inside me finally boiled over. We began arguing more, and I would lash out, fuelled by all the neglect and hurt I had been bottling up.

Dr. Ramani Durvasula once said, "In toxic relationships, anger often becomes a primary mode of communication, fuelled by feelings of inadequacy and neglect." That quote struck a chord with me because it explained exactly how I felt. My anger wasn't just about the arguments—it was about years of feeling unseen, unheard, and undervalued.

During those weeks of binge-watching Netflix, I began to see love in a completely different way. The couples on the screen showed a kind of love that grew over time, one that was built on understanding and real support. They seemed to find happiness in just being together, whether they were exploring something new or enjoying the comfort of everyday life. That kind of love was what I wanted, but it felt so far away. Realising that I had never experienced that in my marriage made me feel confident that my choice to leave in 2021 was the right one. In the days after, I often found myself lost in thought, dreaming about having a partner who truly saw me for who I was. I longed for someone who would understand me, validate my feelings, and encourage my dreams without any judgment. As I thought about my past, I couldn't ignore the years I spent putting on a brave face for the world, hiding the resentment and sadness building up inside me. Those memories reminded me of the exhausting effort to convince myself—and everyone else—that everything was fine, even when my heart felt empty.

Our arguments, especially toward the end, became explosive. They would start small but quickly turn into full-blown toxic arguments, leaving us both feeling hurt and more distant than ever. I can still remember how quickly things could go from calm to chaos, the harsh words we threw at each other widening the gap between us. In those moments, I felt incredibly alone. I yearned for quiet conversations, the kind where couples share their deepest thoughts and fears, but instead, we were stuck in a cycle of blame and anger. Psychologist Dr. Linda Martinez-Lewi once said that narcissism can fuel conflict and lead to outbursts that leave lasting scars, and that hit home for me. Watching Netflix, I noticed how love stories often peel back the layers of a relationship, revealing deeper connections. But when I looked back at my own marriage, peeling back the layers showed me something darker—what I perceived as my husband's growing narcissism. It was like a weight dropped on me, realising I had been living with someone who was potentially emotionally unavailable. I felt trapped in a cycle where I always seemed to be feeding his ego, and when things went wrong, I blamed myself. I realised that gaslighting had become a regular part of our lives; I was constantly questioning whether I was the problem.

This pattern became clear to me after I received 360-degree feedback at work. It was a mirror to my life. At work, I was a confident, strong executive, but at home, I felt invisible, like a shell of who I really was. I had spent so long hiding my own needs that I didn't even know how to express them anymore. Netflix also reminded me that real intimacy isn't just about words; it's about being truly seen and appreciated. While Emmett always encouraged my career, his actions at home told a different story. I felt supported in theory, but in reality, I was suffocating. Over time, I began to lose myself—physically and emotionally. I gained weight, and every time I looked in the mirror, I felt disappointed. How had I let myself get to this point?

From the outside, our life looked perfect. We hosted family events, went on trips, and appeared like a happy couple. But behind closed doors, it was a different story. The weight of unspoken problems and unmet needs was overwhelming. I began to wonder if I would always feel this way: strong and capable at work but lost and empty at home. As I reflected on our life together, it struck me that the love I had been searching for had always felt just out of reach.

I'll never forget sitting at the dining table in July 2024. The evening sunlight poured through the window, bathing the room in a soft glow. Music played quietly in the background, but it only seemed to amplify my thoughts. It was a rare moment of complete honesty with myself. Suddenly, a wave of emotion hit me. It felt like a sharp pain in my chest, and before I knew it, I was crying uncontrollably. Each sob echoed in the quiet room, and I could hardly breathe through the weight of my grief. Those tears brought clarity. I had glimpsed what love could be at times in my relationship with Emmett, but as I sat there, I wondered if it was ever truly love. Was it love or just lust that had pulled us together? As I looked back on our memories, the cracks in our relationship became clearer. The magical moments I used to treasure now seemed tainted by doubt. And then, it hit me: I had never really loved him because I had never truly loved myself. That realisation was painful but honest. What we had shared wasn't real love—it was something else entirely.

This truth felt like lightning, illuminating all the dark corners of my heart that I had ignored for so long. Since starting my journey toward self-love in 2021, I have faced so many challenges. I remember standing in front of the mirror for the first time, following advice from a book I had read. I tried to tell myself, "I love you." But the words wouldn't come. Instead, I felt a deep emptiness, staring at a reflection that seemed like a stranger—someone I didn't believe deserved love. In that moment, I asked myself a question: If I were my own best friend, what would I say to me? The answer hit hard. I had shown myself no compassion. For years, I had been the caretaker, the giver, always putting everyone else first while ignoring my own needs. I held myself to impossible standards, prioritising others' happiness over my own. Somewhere along the way, I had forgotten a fundamental truth: to fully love others, I needed to first embrace and love myself.

Realising this in 2021 was a tough lesson, and the journey to self-acceptance has been far from smooth. There were days when I had breakthroughs, moments of clarity that felt like bright stars in the night. But there were also days when I felt like I was falling into a dark, endless hole. I learned to sit with my feelings, to let myself feel them without judging them. Every time a painful memory or a wave of insecurity came up, I worked on calming myself, gently reminding myself that it was okay to feel lost. Bit by bit, I started to be kinder to myself. It's been a slow process, but every day, I feel a little more complete.

When I look at Emmett now, I see how similar our journeys are in some ways. I suspect that he carries deep wounds—wounds that he hasn't faced. After more than twenty years together, it's clear he's battling his own inner struggles, things he keeps buried inside. I've realised I can't heal those wounds for him. That's a battle he has to fight on his own. But I also know that, like me, he needs to learn to love himself before he can really give or accept love. That truth hurts, but it also feels empowering. Knowing that our struggles may be connected in some way gives me a small sense of hope. Looking back at our marriage, I can't help but question what it was built on. Since we separated, I've uncovered so many lies and deceptions that have clouded my memories of us. It's been a painful process, one that's made me doubt everything I thought I understood about our relationship. I'm not sure he even knows what love really is. We had moments that felt passionate and intense, but now I wonder if those moments were real or just distractions from the emptiness we both carried inside.

As I piece together the memories of our past, I'm more convinced than ever that what we had wasn't real love. We were two hurt people trying to fill our emptiness with each other, instead of building a relationship based on respect and understanding. The more I reflect on it, the more I see that love can't survive without self-acceptance. It's important to acknowledge that this perspective reflects my personal journey, shaped by my experiences and emotions; I must also respect that Emmett may remember certain moments of our lives differently.

Every day, I commit to continuing my journey—not just for myself, but with the hope that one day, I'll find a love that's real. A love that's kind, honest, and built on a deep understanding of who I am and who the other person is. That hope gives me comfort and strength to keep moving forward.

Love as a Mother: Nurturing Bonds and Unconditional Connection

On November 14, 2008, my life changed in ways I never thought possible. When I held my twin boys, Tyson and Zach, for the first time, I felt an overwhelming mix of love, joy, and responsibility. Their tiny fingers wrapped around mine as if sealing a promise for a lifetime of love and connection. From that day on, my journey into motherhood began—a journey that would show me the depths of love, the struggles with control, and the power of being vulnerable.

In the early days, I wanted to be the perfect mother. My sister used to tease me about my hormonal state back then, saying I acted like I was the first mother ever, convinced my way was the only right way. I planned everything about their lives down to the smallest detail, believing that being in control meant I was loving them properly. I planned their meals, decided their activities, and even monitored their friendships. I wanted to protect them from the harshness of the world. When the nannies didn't stick to my plans or forgot to tell me something, I'd get annoyed. Deep down, though, I knew I was struggling with guilt over the long hours I worked and the frequent trips that kept me away from home.

I'll never forget the time one of my sons called me, begging me to come home right away. I had to explain, with a heavy heart, that I was in the United States, and it would take a whole day for me to get back. I tried my best to explain time zones and flights to a toddler, but I could tell he didn't understand. I still remember how I felt when I missed their first steps. They started walking just an hour after I left for a business trip. I was barely at the airport when I got the news during a phone call. Jealousy hit me hard that day. Missing moments like this—and so many other milestones—haunted me.

I tried to be there for their school plays and other events, but I often had to send their nanny, their dad, or a family member in my place. One moment stands out, though: when Zach asked me to come to his school and talk about my job. I didn’t want to let him down, so I said yes, even though I wasn’t sure how to do it. Right before this event, I had gone to India for work and we sponsored a school there as part of a social responsibility project. That experience inspired me. I prepared a simple presentation about my work at a pharmaceutical company that makes consumer healthcare products. I brought enough kids’ toothpaste and mouthwash for every child in his class. I also shared photos of the project in India. I showed the children pictures of a small school where kids sat on the floor while the teacher used a simple blackboard. I told them how we donated Horlicks hot chocolate and biscuits to that school, which, for many kids, was their only meal of the day. I wanted them to appreciate their beautiful school in Surrey and understand that education happens in all kinds of settings. Because I had kept Tyson and Zach in separate classrooms to help them grow as individuals, I had to repeat the presentation for Tyson’s class. As I talked to their classmates, the pride on their faces made all the effort worth it. That day, the children left excited, sharing what they learned with their parents, and I loved seeing my boys so proud.

As the boys grew older, they had a nanny and later an au pair to help care for them. I rarely dropped them off or picked them up from school; that was usually the nanny's job. Even so, every moment I spent with them reminded me how fast time was passing. The guilt of being away so much for work weighed heavily on me. When I was home, I would pour all my energy into being a mother to make up for the time I missed. In doing that, though, I lost sight of myself—not just as a mother, but as a wife and a friend. I often felt lonely.

Their dad wasn't much help. He was like a "helicopter dad," hovering but not really getting involved. He thought that since we had nannies and later an au pair, he didn't need to step in. When he did, it often disrupted the routines I had worked hard to build. The boys thrived on structure, but his sudden involvement threw things into chaos. We argued a lot about our different parenting styles. I knew he loved the boys, but I resented his lack of consistency. He enjoyed socialising with other families, while I preferred to avoid big gatherings. He took the boys to birthday parties most of the time, which I hated attending. Standing around and making small talk with other parents made me uncomfortable. I preferred small playdates with a few parents I felt comfortable with.

One memory stands out clearly. At a school event, I overheard a child ask my sons, "Who is that lady?" My boys proudly said, "That's our mom." But the other child replied, "No, that's not your mom. The other lady is your mom." That comment stung, but I knew it reflected the reality I had created. The boys were usually with their nanny, and I was rarely at these events.

Every decision I made came from wanting to protect them, but I later realised my tight grip often smothered their independence. My fears led me to control their choices and emotions, and even who they were as individuals. I remember the jealousy and insecurity that sometimes clouded my judgment. I wanted to hold onto their love so badly that I acted out of fear instead of genuine affection. Arguments with their father often spiralled into power struggles, where I thought being right made me a better mother. Those moments left me feeling lost and trapped in a cycle of frustration and pain.

As Tyson and Zach entered their teenage years, I started to notice that my control over their lives was slipping away. They were growing into their own people, and with each passing day, I felt the space between us getting bigger. What I once thought of as protecting and loving them now seemed like it might have created walls instead of bridges. I began to wonder if my way of showing love had helped them or held them back.

During this time, I made the tough decision to separate from their father in July 2021. It was a huge change that shook up everything we were used to as a family. But even in the middle of all the upheaval, I felt a small glimmer of hope—a chance to redefine what family meant for us. The separation wasn't easy. It tested my strength and my relationship with the boys. I was dealing with my own emotions while also trying to be their rock. I knew that if I wanted to repair the distance between us, I needed to try something new. That's when I decided to enrol us in a parenting course together, hoping it would help us reconnect and find a new way forward.

The program we joined was called "Executive Functioning Skills: Parents and Children Coaching Program," offered by Connections in Mind UK. It felt like a big leap of faith, but all three of us—Tyson, Zach, and I—were ready to give it a try. The course had ten sessions spread out over several months, and we each worked with our own coach. After each session, we came together to share what we'd learned. Dinner time became a chance to talk openly about our experiences, and slowly, we started to grow closer. One of the first things we tackled was emotional regulation—learning how to handle our feelings in a healthy way. I reflected on how I had reacted in the past, especially during frustrating moments with the boys. I admitted to them that I hadn't always handled those situations well. It was eye-opening to see how some of my behaviours mirrored the things I had struggled with as a child. It wasn't easy to admit, but it felt good to acknowledge it and show them I was trying to change.

Tyson and Zach listened closely as I shared my thoughts, nodding as if they understood. It became clear to all of us that our reactions weren't just personal struggles; they were part of how we interacted as a family. Over time, we started practising calming techniques during conflicts, and I began to see real progress. Each small success felt like a step in the right direction, strengthening our bond. One session focused on time management, which was especially helpful for Tyson. He learned how to set realistic goals and break tasks into smaller steps. I watched proudly as he came up with a plan for his day, including regular breaks as rewards for his hard work. It was incredible to see him taking charge of his own responsibilities.

Another favourite moment was when we completed an assessment to discover our personal values. We gathered at the dinner table, excited to share what we had learned. As we went around, I could see how our values reflected both our individuality and our shared family bond. Tyson shared values that fit his energetic personality, while Zach talked about his thoughtful and caring nature. Listening to them, I saw pieces of myself in their words, but I also saw how unique they were. I shared my own values of compassion and resilience, and together, we had a deep conversation about what mattered most to us as individuals and as a family. That dinner became a turning point. We realised that having different values wasn't a problem—it was something to celebrate. It taught us that our differences made our family stronger, not weaker. We talked about how these differences could help us understand and respect each other more. By the end of the night, I felt closer to the boys than I had in years.

The course brought small but meaningful changes to our family. We started communicating more openly, sharing our struggles without fear and celebrating our progress. The boys began to see my reminders not as nagging but as an effort to provide structure. At the same time, I learned to give them space to figure things out on their own. By the end of the program, I felt incredibly grateful. We had gained new skills and a deeper understanding of each other. Tyson and Zach were stepping up, and becoming more responsible, and I was learning how to support them without taking over. As we wrapped up our final sessions, I looked at my sons and saw a newfound confidence in them. We had faced some tough challenges, but we had come through them stronger and closer as a family. The program wasn't just about learning new skills—it was about rebuilding our connection and creating a future filled with hope and resilience.

A wave of emotions washes over me as I sit here, looking at my nearly sixteen-year-old sons. It feels like just yesterday they were tiny babies in my arms, full of innocence and wonder. Now, they stand before me as young men, each with their own unique personalities, interests, and dreams—a beautiful reflection of the journey we've shared together.

Tyson, my tech-savvy dreamer, is completely absorbed in his love for computers and gaming. I often see him lost in the digital worlds he enjoys so much, forgetting the time as he dives deeper into his passion. He's already built two computers, each one showcasing his talent and creativity. Seeing him so dedicated to something he loves makes me proud and hopeful for his future. Then there's Zach. He's got a sharp mind for math and a creative streak for art and drama—a wonderful mix of logic and imagination. Whether he's solving a tough equation or creating something artistic, he does it with such determination that it amazes me. I admire his resilience and strength, which have grown through the challenges he's faced.

This summer, as an early birthday gift for their upcoming milestone, I took them and four of their closest friends to Tenerife. I thought November might feel too gloomy, so why not celebrate early? Organising the trip was a challenge, but it turned out to be a gift for me too. I was struck by their maturity as we worked through the logistics together. I gave them just two simple rules: save my phone number and never wander off alone. To my surprise—and delight—they stuck to the rules, always moving around in groups of at least three. At the enormous water park, I set myself up under a sun umbrella, keeping a watchful eye as they explored the 40-hectare wonderland. They checked in often, sharing stories about their adventures, their laughter carrying across the park. I played the role of chauffeur, taking them to beaches, go-karting tracks, and even a dolphin-watching trip. It was a whirlwind of activities that left them excited and energised.

Amid all the busyness, there was a comforting rhythm to our days. The house we stayed in had a pool, and it quickly became their favourite spot to play and relax. Of course, they were constantly hungry, but they didn't just wait to be served—they helped out too. They went grocery shopping and pitched in with meal prep. I loved seeing them take charge and make decisions as a team, their bond growing stronger with each moment. As the evenings rolled around, I'd retreat to my space, giving them room to enjoy their independence. They stayed up late, laughing and bonding, while I found peace knowing they were happy and safe. When we returned home to Switzerland, I felt a sense of achievement. The trip had been a success, with no mishaps, and the boys were genuinely grateful. Seeing how much they appreciated the experience filled me with pride.

When it comes to their academics, I don't worry much. They're both thriving in their own ways. I've always encouraged them to follow their interests, celebrating their differences rather than comparing them. It's heartwarming to see how they support each other, combining their strengths to overcome challenges.

Co-parenting hasn't been without its difficulties, especially after changes in our family dynamic. But I'm proud of how well we've managed to protect the boys from any negativity. Every Sunday, they switch homes—one week with me, one week with their dad. We've worked hard to prioritise their needs, adapting our schedules to keep things peaceful. It's a delicate balance, but we've made it work, and the boys remain happy and secure.

The love I share with my boys has grown and evolved over the years. It's now rooted in mutual respect and acceptance. I'm no longer just their caregiver; I'm their supporter, cheering them on as they grow into the men they're becoming. Our home is a place of openness and trust, where we celebrate each other's successes—big or small—and stand together through tough times. I've also learned that being vulnerable can be a strength. By sharing my struggles with them, we've deepened our connection, creating a bond that helps us all grow as individuals. As Tyson and Zach approach adulthood, I feel grateful for the lessons we've learned together.

This journey of motherhood has shown me that love has the power to transform. It heals, inspires empathy, and creates a safe space for growth. As I embrace this new chapter with my boys, I find comfort in knowing that our bond will only grow stronger. Love is the foundation that guides us through life's challenges and keeps us grounded. I'm excited for the adventures ahead, confident that together we can face anything with strength and grace.

Love Among Family and Friends: The Strength of Cherished Connections

South African Chapter: Connections and Growth

When I look back on my journey of love among my family and friends, I see how often I came at it from a place of fear and insecurity. In those early years, I craved love like a thirsty person looking for water in a desert. I held on tightly to the people I loved, thinking that if I didn't let go, I could avoid feeling abandoned.

Growing up in a big family with ten siblings, I spent most of my childhood with the youngest four of us. We formed a close bond that became my foundation. As my older siblings got married or moved away for work, our family's dynamic changed, leaving my younger siblings as my main companions. In this small circle, I learned what friendship really means. It wasn't always smooth—we often argued and were territorial about the little we had, leading to fights over belongings and jealousy. Still, the core of my friendships came from the lessons I learned within my family. The loyalty, trust, and love we shared as siblings set the tone for the kind of friends I wanted. I looked for people who valued support and honesty, and I realised that good friendships, like strong families, need communication and a willingness to stick together through tough times.

My first friendships were with kids in the neighbourhood, where we played outside on the street. My first best friend, Vanessa, has been in my life ever since. Even though she now lives in New Zealand and I'm in Switzerland, we've stayed in touch. We grew up together and shared many moments, like when I was her bridesmaid. We don't talk as often now, but we still exchange WhatsApp messages and birthday wishes. Music keeps us connected, as Vanessa often sends songs that remind us of our childhood memories.

Then there was the Kazmer family, our neighbours. Clint, who was born in the same month as me, became a close friend. I would often escape the busyness of my house by hopping over the fence to their place. Clint's mom, Aunty Yvonne, taught me how to bake, and I still think fondly of those times kneading dough and frosting cakes. My first trip abroad was to visit the Kazmers in Australia after a breakup. That trip helped me heal and reflect before starting my job at a South African retailer. Although I've lost touch with Clint and Aunty Yvonne, I stay connected to their sister, Bronwyn, through WhatsApp. This year, I hosted Bronwyn and her family at my holiday cottage in Devon for Christmas and welcomed them to my home in Switzerland a few weeks later.

Another important friendship was with the Thomas family. Noelene, who was older than me, became a close friend, and I was honoured to become the godmother of her daughter Camille. Even though we live far apart now, we stay in touch with occasional visits and birthday messages. Our long phone calls feel effortless, like no time has passed. I especially enjoyed their recent visit to Switzerland, where we shared stories and connected over Camille's experiences.

As I reflect on these friendships, I see that while my early connections were meaningful, the relationships I built later in life have been deeper and more rewarding, reflecting how I've grown as a person.

Family relationships, however, have been more challenging. It's true what they say—you often fight with those closest to you. Growing up in South Africa, my sibling relationships weren't always healthy. Insecurity made me act out, and my need to hold on to love sometimes led me to pick fights over small things. Ironically, I often pushed away the very people I wanted to be close to. After each argument, I felt lonely and misunderstood, retreating into my thoughts and doubting if I deserved love at all.

But one relationship has been a constant source of strength: my sister Dawn. Our bond is truly special and hard to put into words. From the start, she made me feel safe and never judged. I could talk to her about anything, and she always listened with an open heart. Dawn has been there for me during my hardest times, lifting me up when I felt lost. She's been my confidante, my cheerleader, and my safe place. When I felt overwhelmed, her presence gave me comfort. She's seen me at my most vulnerable and still loved me without hesitation. My love for her goes beyond words. It's a deep understanding that doesn't need explanation. Even when my words hurt her, she stayed by my side, always showing me unconditional love. This, I believe, is the essence of true love—staying strong through life's ups and downs and growing closer because of it.

As the author Anna Quindlen beautifully said, "Sisters are different flowers from the same garden." This quote perfectly describes our relationship. Despite our differences, we are deeply connected. Together, we've built a bond that is strong and unshakable, and it continues to enrich my life every day.

London Chapter: Connections and Growth

When I moved to London in 2002, I had no idea how important Emma would become in my life. From the moment we met, she became like a guide, helping me navigate the complex dynamics of the Munyoro family. Emma welcomed me into her world with open arms, and over the years, our connection grew through visits, shared laughter, and memorable family moments. She became more than just a cousin-in-law—she became like a sister to me.

One of the most important moments she was there for me was when my twin boys were born. Emma rushed to the hospital, bringing comfort during one of the biggest changes in my life. I still remember how her face lit up when she held my boys for the first time. It wasn't just about the arrival of my children—it was a reminder of how strong our bond was. She was there to share in my joy and offer reassurance as I adjusted to motherhood. One memory that stands out is a chaotic Christmas morning. I was exhausted from sleepless nights and trying to prepare the turkey. Emma and I ended up laughing hysterically as we tried to find the giblets hidden inside the bird. That moment of shared laughter lightened the stress of motherhood and reminded me how wonderful it is to have someone by your side. When Emma moved to my village, it felt like a blessing. Having her close meant we could spend more time together, from casual coffee dates to deep conversations about life. Her laughter and support turned ordinary days into cherished moments.

After my marriage ended, Emma's support was unwavering. She listened to me vent about my frustrations with Emmett, my ex-husband, without judging me. Her ability to stay neutral and offer thoughtful advice was exactly what I needed. She reminded me of my strength and made me feel less alone. I'll always be grateful for her presence during that difficult time—for being that rare family member who stood by me and my boys, no matter what. Sharing heartbreak and healing with Emma has made me even more grateful for her in ways I struggle to fully express. She knows what it's like to deal with loss and how hard it can be to move forward, and this shared understanding has helped us support each other. When I felt weighed down by the struggles of being a single mom or the emotional strain of divorce, Emma reminded me that I wasn't alone. We worked through life's challenges together, finding strength in our friendship and creating a safe place where we could be open about our feelings. When things felt tough, Emma's kindness reminded me of the strength we both have. Our friendship has become a place of comfort where we can share our worries and celebrate our wins. Every conversation, laugh, and moment we share feels so special because they've brought us closer.

As life goes on, I feel so lucky to have Emma in my life. She shows me what family really means—someone who sticks with you through everything and offers love and understanding when you need it most. I look forward to all the future moments we'll share, knowing we'll face whatever comes together, supported by the bond we've built.

Thinking about my time with Emmett's family in the UK brings up some mixed feelings. On the one hand, we shared many moments together, but on the other, it often felt like our relationship didn't grow as deeply as I'd hoped. After Emmett and I split, there was a clear distance between us that left me wishing for stronger connections. It wasn't that anyone meant to hurt me, but the relationships often felt shallow. Family events were especially hard—I would try to make the gatherings warm and welcoming, but I often found myself cleaning up alone after everyone left. Their laughter would still echo, reminding me of the closeness I longed for but didn't feel.

One exception was Emmett's aunt, Aunty Isabel. She stood by me when my marriage was falling apart, offering kindness and support without judgment. It broke my heart when her relationship with me caused tension with Emmett. He believed his family's loyalty should always lie with him, even if that meant pushing her away. I wanted to keep her living in one of our homes, but Emmett insisted she move out, which left me feeling helpless. Watching her pack her things and leave to live with her daughter was heartbreaking, especially since Emma was also going through her own divorce at the time. It felt so unfair to see Aunty Isabel, who had once been such a strong support for Emmett, caught up in the aftermath of our separation. I couldn't understand why Emmett, who claimed to love and respect her, would put her in such a painful position. Trying to navigate his behaviour was exhausting, and I knew stepping in could have legal consequences because of our separation agreement.

These challenges taught me a lot about family and the lessons that come with those relationships. Ending a 20-year marriage was my choice, but I never expected it would be met with such emotional distance. After I left, the silence from Emmett's family was deafening. Many of them visited him in Switzerland to offer support, but they didn't reach out to me, which deepened my sense of isolation. Despite the pain, I've learned to value the connections that matter most. I've decided to focus my energy on relationships that give back the love and effort I put into them. I'll always cherish the good memories and let go of what no longer serves me, hoping this brings me peace and fulfilment.

While living in London, my relationship with my family in South Africa has grown stronger, even though we're so far apart. I make it a point to visit them every year, spending time with my many siblings and their families. These trips are always busy and tiring as we move from Johannesburg to Durban and Cape Town, but they remind me how important it is to stay connected.

I was overjoyed to bring nearly all my siblings to visit me in London. They couldn't afford the trip themselves, so I felt fulfilled being able to sponsor their journeys using the air miles I'd earned from work travel. While they were in London, I even took them on a trip to another European country, creating memories we'll all treasure forever.

One relationship that means a lot to me is with Lorraine, my brother Keith's ex-wife, and their two daughters, Rozanne and Arlene. I'm honoured to have been part of their lives, especially attending both daughters' weddings as the only family member present. Sadly, our connection faded after Keith and Lorraine divorced. For years, my family lost touch with Lorraine and the girls, and Keith distanced himself from his children as he dealt with his own struggles. When Keith returned home years later, gravely ill and without medical benefits, I felt overwhelmed with worry. The local hospital couldn't help him, and as his youngest sister, I couldn't stand by and do nothing. From London, I arranged for him to be treated at a private hospital in South Africa.

I called Lorraine to tell her about Keith's condition. I said, "Lorraine, I promised not to contact speak to the girls about Keith, but you may have to now. He's very sick, and we don't know what will happen." She decided to tell Rozanne and Arlene, who travelled from Pretoria to Durban, to see him. It felt like the universe was working to bring our family back together. Keith got to reconnect with his daughters after 20 years, and he even survived, living three more years sober and rebuilding his bond with them. Keith passed away on New Year's Day three years later, but during those years, our family grew closer to Lorraine, Rozanne, and Arlene. I'm grateful that being able to pay for Keith's care not only saved his life at the time but also gave him a chance to repair relationships that meant so much.

Over the years, I've built many friendships in South Africa and London. Each one has added something special to my life. This chapter doesn't include every relationship I've had, but it gives a glimpse of the ones that shaped me. Whether those friendships lasted a long time or not, I'm thankful for all the memories and lessons they brought.

Switzerland Chapter: Connections and Growth

During my time in Switzerland, I discovered how relationships can grow and deepen in meaningful ways. The peaceful beauty of the country, with its stunning landscapes, became the backdrop for my personal growth. It was here that I started to truly understand what it means to love without fear or expectation. This lesson came slowly, shaped by powerful experiences and conversations that challenged how I saw the world. Once I allowed myself to embrace love in its purest form, I felt a shift within me. I spent time reflecting on my insecurities, facing them, and letting myself grow.

This chapter of my life marked the start of forming the deep connections I had always longed for. Four amazing women—Nicole, Emily, Christine, and Bonita—each played a key role in this transformation. Nicole helped me see parts of myself I had forgotten or ignored. She believed in my potential, even when I doubted it, and encouraged me to be open and vulnerable. She showed me how sharing our stories, both happy and painful, can create strong connections. Through her, I realised that our experiences shape who we are and help us relate to others. Emily, Bonita, and Christine have been my anchors during the hardest moments of my growth. They've listened without judgment, offered kind advice, and reminded me that I'm not alone. Their support has been a powerful reminder of the strength of friendship and sisterhood. They've shown me that love can help us get through even the toughest times. Each of them has made my life richer in ways that are hard to describe, and I will always be grateful for the bonds we've built. Together, we've created a strength that lifts us up and helps us face life with courage and grace.

Nicole

My friendship with Nicole started in a way that felt like fate, as though the universe brought us together at the perfect moment. It was during the uncertain days of COVID-19 when I received a LinkedIn message from her. She was curious about my move to Switzerland and wanted to connect. She thought we might be able to learn from each other. Even though I had never used social media this way, something told me to accept her invitation. During our first virtual meeting, we connected in a way that felt effortless. The conversation flowed naturally, and it felt like we had known each other for years. I finished the call feeling amazed, thinking, "That was different." Talking to someone so genuine and positive was refreshing during such a difficult time.

A few days later, I received a package at my door. It was Nicole's book, along with a note that said: *"Dear Rochelle, It was a joy and an honour to get to know you and feel your authenticity radiate way beyond the limitations of meeting virtually. When a company gets you, they invite vision, clarity, change, wind energy, and fast dynamic growth. I can't wait to meet you in person. —Nicole Kilchberg, September 2, 2020"*

Her words struck a chord. Even though we had only spoken for an hour, she had seen something in me that I hadn't fully seen in myself. She recognised my potential and essence in a way that felt profound. Nicole wasn't just anyone—she was an executive coach and a published author, yet she spoke to me as a friend who believed in me deeply. Encouraged by her words, I started reading her book, *How to Develop the Authentic Leader in You.* The book felt like it was speaking directly to me, each chapter making me think about authenticity, vulnerability, and aligning with my values. For the first time, I felt truly seen, and it inspired me to reflect on who I am and who I want to be.

As our relationship grew, I asked Nicole to help with a leadership development project at work. She became a valuable part of the process, especially through the 360-degree leadership assessments she facilitated for our executive team. These assessments opened my eyes and made me confront important questions: Who am I? What do I believe in? How can I lead in an authentic way when the world often demands conformity?

Our professional relationship soon turned into a close friendship. We talked about everything—not just work, but personal struggles, dreams, and victories. She encouraged me to share my challenges and celebrate my progress, no matter how small. In her presence, I felt safe exploring my identity and facing my fears. Nicole became more than just a coach or colleague; she became a trusted friend. Her constant support gave me the strength to follow my passions and redefine my goals. Looking back, I feel so grateful for that first message that brought us together. It turned into a connection that changed my life. In a world where real relationships can feel rare, I treasure our bond. It's built on authenticity, respect, and the desire to help each other grow.

I was also thrilled when Nicole and her husband, Han, invited me to work with their Foundation. This foundation focuses on sponsoring the education of young indigenous leaders in the Amazon, a mission that deeply aligns with my values.

Our journey to the Amazon was life-changing. We explored lush landscapes and connected with vibrant communities. The people we met shared stories and wisdom that bridged the gap between our worlds. Their connection to the land and their knowledge of sustainable living made me rethink my own relationship with nature.We saw the many challenges they face—deforestation, climate change, and threats to their lands. These experiences showed me how critical education is in helping young indigenous leaders protect their communities and environment. The foundation's goal isn't just academic success but also preserving cultural identity and empowering these leaders to create meaningful change. This collaboration with Nicole and Han deepened my understanding of how connected we all are. It inspired me to advocate for indigenous rights and environmental protection. Working with the foundation has been a reminder of the importance of creating a better future for our planet and its diverse cultures.

Meeting Nicole felt like a gift from the universe, arriving when I needed it most. Our friendship has been filled with shared joy and support, and she has helped me grow into the person I'm meant to be. Today, I can say with confidence that I love who I am. The essence of who I've always been is finally shining through, after years of hiding under scars and fears. Every experience has been part of this journey toward self-discovery and authenticity. Nicole lit a spark within me that was waiting to burn bright. Now, I live with love in my heart, and that love flows into everything I do. Every day, I feel closer to my purpose and my true self. My friendship with Nicole is more than just a story; it's proof of the magic that can happen when we connect deeply with others.

Bonita

I first met Bonita in South Africa in 2001. She was a vibrant, free spirit who joined a top 10 global fast-moving consumer goods company, where I had already been working since 1999. From the moment we met, there was an instant connection, like we'd known each other forever. We quickly became friends, sharing laughs, long chats, and dreams about the future. Our group of friends felt like a family, a warm and supportive bubble in the middle of our busy work lives.

But life took me in a new direction. I got an exciting job offer at the company's headquarters in London. While I was excited, I also felt nervous about leaving. I carried Bonita's friendship with me, holding it close like a piece of home. A few years later, Bonita moved to London, too, chasing her own dreams. I thought we'd pick up right where we left off, but things didn't turn out that way. Life in London was fast-paced and hectic. My job consumed most of my time, with endless meetings and constant travel. The fun, carefree friendship we once had started to feel distant. I missed our spontaneous coffee breaks, laughing until our stomachs hurt, and just being in each other's company. Even though I was focused on my career, I couldn't help but feel a little empty without the bond we once had.

Then came Bonita's wedding in Hannover, Germany. It was a bright and joyful moment in the middle of our busy lives. The day was full of love and happiness, with an energy that was contagious. Watching Bonita and Sebastian exchange vows filled me with joy. That night was magical—we danced until the early hours of the morning, lost in the music and the moment. It reminded me that, despite the distance and changes in our lives, our friendship still had the power to bring so much joy.

Life changed again when Bonita became a mom. Her daughter Phoebe arrived, and I watched her step into motherhood with strength and grace. It was a beautiful but demanding chapter for her. Our visits became less frequent as we both got swept up in our busy lives. Bonita, who had always been so carefree and spontaneous, was now focused on sleepless nights, baby milestones, and the deep love that comes with being a parent.

In 2008, my twin boys, Tyson and Zach, were born, adding a new layer to my life. Then, in 2012, Bonita and Sebastian welcomed their twin daughters, Francesca and Kiara. Motherhood brought even more joy but also made it harder for us to keep in touch the way we used to. We were both so busy raising our kids—diaper changes, playdates, and the constant surprises that come with little ones. I missed our deep conversations and long chats but knew this was a special and exhausting time for both of us.

till, I held onto the little moments we could share: a quick coffee, a short message full of laughter, or just knowing we were there for each other. Our friendship had changed, but I hoped we could continue to support each other as we navigated this new chapter of life.

In 2015, Bonita made the hard decision to move back to South Africa. Saying goodbye was bittersweet. I felt sad to see her go but hopeful we'd find ways to stay connected. Even though we were now on different continents, our bond stayed strong. We leaned on each other, using video calls, heartfelt messages, and rare visits when I travelled to South Africa to keep our connection alive.

By late 2022, Bonita reached out for help with a project that needed my professional skills. This brought us back together in an unexpected way. As we worked together, our conversations became deeper, moving beyond work to our personal lives. We talked about our struggles, fears, and victories, and those talks felt like a healing balm for our friendship.

I remember one conversation where I told Bonita, "Everything happens for a reason." It felt like the universe had brought us back together at just the right time. We were both facing challenges in our own lives, but through our renewed connection, we found strength and purpose. Every story we shared and every honest moment brought us closer, giving our friendship a fresh start.

It felt like we'd entered a new chapter. We embraced honesty and celebrated vulnerability, which made our bond even stronger. I felt grateful for the chance to reconnect and grow together. Even though life was still busy, our friendship became a sanctuary—a place where we could truly be ourselves.

Now that Bonita and her family have moved back to Europe and are living in Germany, it's been easier to visit and spend time together. This has made me even more thankful for the journey we've shared. Despite all the twists and turns, our friendship has only grown stronger. Bonita isn't just a friend; she's a kindred spirit. Our connection has stood the test of time, reminding me that true friendship can survive anything, becoming even richer and deeper along the way.

Emily

I first met Emily in February 2016, on a clear, cold winter day that felt full of possibilities. I was interviewing candidates for an HR coordinator job at a consumer health company. When she walked into the room, she brought a sense of warmth and light with her. She seemed confident but also a little unsure, like she carried something special inside her that she hadn't fully realised yet. I remember thinking how genuine she seemed. From that moment, she stood out to me.

After all the interviews, I knew she was the right choice. She joined my team in March, and over the following months, her energy and enthusiasm changed our workplace. Her laughter became a regular part of the office, easing the usual stress of work. Emily had this amazing way of making everyone feel important and appreciated. I loved our conversations; she had a way of telling stories that made me laugh and sharing thoughts that inspired me.

But life took an unexpected turn. By September 2016, I had a new opportunity that I couldn’t pass up. The decision to leave the consumer health company was tough because I wasn’t just leaving a job; I was leaving the start of a friendship with someone I really believed in. I sat down with Emily, nervous about how she’d take the news. “I’m really sorry to be leaving,” I said, trying to keep my voice steady. “But I see so much potential in you. If you’re interested, I can hire you as my executive assistant at the pharmaceutical company. From there, I’ll help you grow into other HR roles when they open up.” I wasn’t sure what she’d say, but she agreed right away. It felt like a leap of faith for both of us.

In October 2016, she joined me at the pharmaceutical company, and I got to see her shine in this new role. Emily’s energy and excitement for the work were contagious, and I loved seeing her thrive. Less than a year later, an HR role opened up. I encouraged her to go for it, but I wasn’t her direct boss anymore. I wanted her to earn it on her own. “You’ve got this, Emily,” I told her. “You’re more than ready for this. Trust yourself.” She applied, got the job, and I couldn’t have been prouder. Watching her grow from a newcomer into a confident professional was incredible.

As Emily moved into new roles, I gave her space to grow on her own. I wasn’t directly involved anymore, but I admired how much energy and passion she brought to her work. By August 2019, I felt she was ready to stand completely on her own. When I left the pharmaceutical company, it was bittersweet, knowing I was leaving behind someone I had so much faith in.

In early 2020, I had a chance to recommend her for another job at a top five Japanese pharmaceutical company, where I'd been working since the previous September. My colleague needed someone with Emily's skills, and I immediately thought of her. I made it clear that my recommendation was based on her abilities, not our history, and I wouldn't be involved in the hiring process. I wanted her to succeed on her own. She joined the pharmaceutical company in May 2020, and it felt good to know I'd been part of her journey again.

When I decided to leave the company in September 2020, I joked with her, "This is the last time I'm recommending you for anything because it's time for you to make your own way." She laughed and said, "Well, it wouldn't look good for you if I keep following you and end up with another awful boss!" Her humour always made me smile.

What started as a professional relationship grew into something much deeper. Emily worked directly for me for just a few months at the consumer health company and less than a year at the pharmaceutical company, but our connection turned into a real friendship. There was something about her that drew me in. She reminded me of a younger version of myself—full of potential but sometimes held back by self-doubt. I saw a spark in her that made me want to help her see just how amazing she could be.

Emily's honesty and openness really stood out when she went through a tough time in her personal life. She decided to end her marriage, a choice that took incredible strength. I admired her courage as she faced this challenge and opened up about her feelings. It brought us even closer. Supporting her through that time taught me a lot about resilience and vulnerability. In fact, her strength helped me prepare for my own struggles.

Both of our ex-husbands had similar difficult traits, which created a unique bond between us. Emily's support during my own tough times meant so much to me. We became a source of strength for each other, helping one another face our fears and doubts. It felt like we were sisters in some ways—guiding and uplifting each other.

Emily has a rare gift for connecting with people. She's not afraid to show her emotions, and her openness makes her truly special. She helped me feel comfortable being vulnerable, too, something I'd avoided in the past. Through her, I rediscovered parts of myself that I'd pushed aside.

Looking back, I'm amazed at how our professional connection turned into such a meaningful friendship. Emily taught me that being vulnerable isn't a weakness; it's a kind of strength. By helping her in her career, I ended up finding a deeper connection with her and with myself. Our friendship is built on shared experiences, respect, and a deep understanding of each other. It's a bond that has helped both of us grow and heal. We've shared laughter and tears, supported each other through challenges, and celebrated our victories. Together, we've created a friendship that's not just about helping each other professionally but about being there for each other in life. And that's something I'll always treasure.

Christine

I first met Christine in 2006 during the interview process at Global FMCG Company. My task was to prepare to hand over my role to her, which felt a bit daunting. But the moment I saw her, I was drawn in. Christine had a quiet confidence that was magnetic, and when she spoke, it was like listening to something beautifully composed. She shared her vision with passion and clarity, talking about how important it was to help people grow and make a real difference at work. Although we only worked together briefly—since I moved to another role and then a different company by 2008—Christine left a deep impression on me. I felt a connection with her that stayed with me long after that initial meeting.

In 2010, I had the chance to bring Christine into my new company, B2B Manufacturing. It felt like a rare opportunity to reconnect and work together again. However, I had my doubts. B2B Manufacturing was much smaller than the consumer goods company, and I wasn't sure if she would take the leap. I felt nervous, hopeful, and unsure all at once. But our shared passion for developing others and creating meaningful work drew her in. When Christine said yes to the offer, I was thrilled. It felt like the universe had given me a gift by bringing us back together.

Working with Christine turned out to be one of the best experiences of my career. She challenged me in ways I hadn't expected, inspiring us to dig deeper into our work and aim higher. Christine had a talent for making people strive for excellence. She never accepted anything less than our best, and her commitment to quality was incredible. I soaked up her insights like a sponge. Time spent working with Christine wasn't just about getting things done; it was about building something meaningful together, based on trust and a shared vision.

Over time, our bond grew stronger. We worked long hours, but we also shared personal moments that deepened our friendship. At the time, I was a mother to toddler twin boys, a phase of life that was both joyful and overwhelming. I remember when my team, including Christine, came to my home to meet my sons. Those visits were short but incredibly special. Watching Christine interact with my boys was heartwarming. She had such a natural connection with children, and her laughter filled my home with happiness that stayed long after she left.

Christine is one of those rare people who gives so much of herself, often putting others first. Her care and generosity were evident in everything she did. When I moved on to the consumer health company, Christine continued to support me. She often visited, bringing little gifts for my boys that lit up their faces. She was like a steady presence in my life, offering advice and encouragement. Whether we talked about work, parenting, or life in general, her wisdom was always practical and thoughtful.

As the years passed, I found more opportunities to work with Christine. She became a coach, and her guidance proved invaluable, not just for my teams at consumer health company but also at one of the top five Japanese pharmaceutical company. I had complete faith in her abilities and knew how much of a difference she could make.

Christine became a regular guest at my home. She celebrated my boys' birthdays with us, helping me throw their parties and sharing in the laughter and cake. These moments of connection were like reminders of the family we had built through friendship and respect. No matter what was happening in our lives, our relationship remained strong and full of joy.

Then came the difficult moment when I had to tell Christine that I was moving to Switzerland. Breaking the news felt heavy, and I imagined she must have felt the same. We both knew things would change, though we couldn't predict how. Even so, Christine stayed by my side during that transition. She helped me pack, her laughter easing the sadness of leaving. We shared stories and memories as we prepared for the next chapter of our lives. Her support during that time meant the world to me.

Once I settled in Switzerland, I faced challenges I hadn't expected. The beauty of the mountains and lakes sometimes felt at odds with the struggles I was going through inside. I often felt isolated, grappling with emotions I hadn't shared with anyone before. Christine was the first person I opened up to about my troubled marriage. Her response was exactly what I needed—kind and without judgment. She listened patiently, offering support and words of comfort that helped me through some of my darkest moments.

Our conversations grew even deeper over time. Christine began to share her own challenges with me, and this mutual openness brought us closer. It wasn't just about me anymore; we were both leaning on each other, sharing our truths and navigating life's hurdles together. This new level of honesty strengthened our bond in ways I hadn't imagined.

I often feel honoured to be one of Christine's closest friends. In many ways, it feels like our relationship is unique, maybe even stronger than the bonds she shares with her own family. I treasure our connection deeply. I think back fondly to the time she visited me in Switzerland, where we spent peaceful afternoons together, simply enjoying each other's company. Those moments felt like a sanctuary, a reminder of how easily we understood each other.

I'm deeply grateful for Christine and the journey we've shared. She has been a source of growth, inspiration, and unwavering support. As I look back on our friendship, I feel nothing but appreciation and look forward to all the memories still to come. I know that wherever life takes us, Christine will always hold a special place in my heart.

In conclusion

As I sit here reflecting on this chapter, I see how far I've come in facing the fears that used to control how I behaved in relationships with my family and friends. It hasn't been an easy journey, but it's taught me to value the unique qualities of the people I care about. Instead of feeling threatened by their individuality, I've learned to celebrate it.

When I was a child, the connections I had with others were based on the comfort of being familiar with each other. But as life took us to different parts of the world, those relationships didn't get the chance to deepen in the ways I hoped. It didn't mean the love was gone—it just meant our relationships changed in ways I didn't fully understand back then.

Later, when I lived in London, I poured so much energy into my career and raising my family that my friendships often revolved around work. Life was busy, and I ended up neglecting many relationships. Even so, I'm thankful for the lasting bonds I've kept with people like Bonita, Emily, and Christine. These friendships have endured, growing and changing over time and distance.

Moving to Switzerland marked a big turning point for me. It was here that I found something new in my friendships. I allowed myself to be real and honest, letting go of the need to hide parts of my life. This honesty became a two-way street, and my relationships grew deeper and more meaningful. New friendships, like the one I've built with Nicole, brought incredible richness to my life. Meanwhile, my bonds with Bonita, Emily, and Christine became stronger in ways I had always wished for. In Switzerland, I found the kind of connections I'd been searching for my whole life—ones that go beyond family ties and blossom into something much deeper, filled with unconditional love. This new understanding brought me peace, which I had been missing for years. I learned how to truly listen instead of reacting and how to offer support instead of trying to control. My relationships became a source of joy rather than a cause for worry, and I grew to appreciate the people in my life even more.

Even the dynamics with my sisters changed. I treasure the memories of the days we spent together at my Benguela Cove home in April 2024, where we laughed and shared stories without the tension that had once affected us. Those moments felt warm and comforting, like we were wrapped in a sense of belonging. I realised it was important to accept what each relationship had to offer and to give love without expecting anything in return. It meant allowing space for all of us to be ourselves.

As I kept growing, I found balance in my relationships. Love became less about holding on tightly and more about sharing and letting go. I discovered that I could cherish someone deeply while also giving them the freedom to be who they truly are. The respect and acceptance I cultivated made all the difference. I stopped feeling the need to monitor every interaction, trusting instead that those who cared about me would stay in my life.

Looking back, I see how far I've come—from living in fear to finding freedom. Now, I value the relationships I have with my family and friends, knowing that real love thrives when it's not weighed down by expectations or attachment. As Maya Angelou so wisely said, "I sustain myself with the love of family." It's a love that lifts me up and encourages me, giving me the strength to face life's ups and downs. In this love, I've found not only strength but also the beauty of true, cherished connections.

Nourishing Love: Cultivating a Relationship with What I Feed My Body

When I was growing up, the kitchen was the heart of our home. It was a warm, bright space that always smelled amazing, filled with the scents of vegetables from our garden and, on special days, roasted meat. My mom had a gift for turning simple ingredients into delicious meals. I can still picture her picking fresh veggies and herbs, her hands moving so smoothly, as if she were pulling out the best flavours from everything. Cooking for her wasn't just about making food; it was something special, almost like an art. And when she brought home chicken or beef, it felt like a big deal—a celebration. Food wasn't just something to eat; it was her way of showing love, a kind of care that made us feel safe and happy. As Gary Chapman says in his book, acts of service, like cooking for your family, are a powerful way to show love (Chapman, 1992). I learned early on that a warm bowl of soup or a plate of my favourite dish, Samp and Beans, could make a bad day better. I remember my mom pouring soup into our bowls, each spoonful filled with her love. The warmth of the broth seemed to chase away all the little pains of childhood, whether it was a scraped knee or a harsh word from a sibling. Those meals were more than just food; they were moments of connection, even when we didn't talk much. In that kitchen, I felt happy and cared for, and food became something I looked forward to.

With ten siblings, it's no surprise that food was a big part of our family gatherings. I can still taste the meals my older sisters made—hearty stews on cold winter nights and fresh, flavorful salads in the summer. Preparing meals together was like a dance, with everyone playing their part. Food was how we celebrated, how we bonded, and even how we healed from tough times. I loved the laughter, the teasing, and the playful arguments over who had made the best dish that day.

But as I grew older, the weight of my past started to catch up with me. The pain I had buried deep inside began to surface, shaping how I acted in ways I didn't fully understand. I felt a constant need to prove myself, driven by an endless hunger for approval. When I moved to London and Switzerland to work in the corporate world, food became my comfort. I often found myself longing for my mother's kitchen—the safety and love it symbolised—during stressful moments at work. Without realising it, my stress started to control how I ate. When the pressure got too much, I turned to food for comfort, especially dishes that reminded me of home. But as my career took off, my eating habits spiralled out of control. The demands of my job—long flights, late meetings—meant I often ate at odd hours or skipped meals entirely. I remember sitting in business class on long flights, eating fancy meals and sipping champagne, trying to convince myself I had everything under control. But deep down, I felt lost. Those big dinners with leadership teams felt like brief distractions, a way to escape the constant feeling that I wasn't good enough.

Then motherhood arrived—a beautiful but overwhelming chapter of my life. I wanted to nourish my children the way my mother had nourished me, putting love into every meal. I imagined creating the same warm, happy environment where food brought joy and connection. But balancing a demanding executive job with parenting left me little time for self-care. I often skipped meals, caught up in the endless cycle of work and family responsibilities. When I did eat, it was usually my kids' leftovers or whatever I could grab quickly.

In those early years, meals felt lonely. They were nothing like the big family feasts I used to love. My husband and I were often apart, both busy with our careers. When I was home, I would take over from the nanny, rushing through the evening routine. My kids ate early, their laughter filling the house, while I worked late, eating quickly and without joy. The kitchen, once a place of warmth and connection, became just another room where I hurried through my tasks. I missed the joy of eating together as a family—the laughter, the stories, and the way we used to connect over meals. Instead, I found myself eating alone, listening to the sound of cutlery on plates. Each meal reminded me of what I was missing: the warmth of togetherness and the simple pleasure of sharing food with loved ones.

Over time, the stress and loneliness started to show in my body. At first, the changes were small, but they added up. I went from a small to a medium, and then to a large, and each time I had to buy new clothes, it felt like a reminder of my struggles. After I had my twin boys in 2008, I began wearing clothes that hid my growing belly and thighs. I leaned toward dark colours, especially black, hoping they would make me feel less noticeable. But no matter how much I tried to cover up, I couldn't escape the shame I felt. My body became a source of constant discomfort, and I felt judged everywhere I went.

In those quiet moments of reflection, I often thought about my childhood kitchen—the smells, the warmth, and the love it held. I missed sitting around the table with my family, sharing food that nourished not just our bodies but our spirits. Now, food felt like a chore, a reminder of how far I had drifted from the joy I once knew. Through this whirlwind, I later realised that my relationship with food had become distorted. What was once a source of comfort had turned into a way to escape my stress. As Roxane Gay writes in *Hunger: A Memoir of (My) Body*, "Food is a complex part of my experience. It is both a source of comfort and a source of anxiety, a way to deal with my feelings and a reminder of how I feel about myself" I was stuck in a cycle of unhealthy eating habits, and the simple act of taking care of myself had become difficult.

In December 2023, I shared a heartfelt lunch with my dear friends Han and Nicole, who had just returned from a life-changing health retreat with Dr. Fuhrman in San Diego, California. Nicole, my close friend and mentor, has been a guiding influence in my life since 2020, and seeing her vibrant energy after the retreat filled me with happiness. As they spoke with passion about their experiences, I could see how much both of them had changed, especially Han, who had courageously stopped taking his medications. Their journey wasn't just about food; it was a testament to a fresh start in life. Listening to them talk about their time at the retreat, I felt inspired. Nicole's commitment to health and wellness had always inspired me, but seeing the real impact it had on her and Han deepened my admiration. Han's transformation was particularly moving—his decision to embrace this new lifestyle and take back control of his health was truly amazing. The way they spoke about the powerful knowledge they gained and the supportive community they found at the retreat made me realise that such big changes are possible when someone is dedicated to self-care and well-being.

Their experiences sparked something inside me, reminding me of the importance of taking care of not just our bodies but also our minds. The deep admiration I felt for their dedication to health and the inspiration they provided pushed me to begin my own journey toward change. I left that lunch not only uplifted by their stories but also motivated to explore what transformation could look like in my own life, inspired by their strength and resilience.

In summary, this is what I learned from that nourishing lunch. Dr. Joel Fuhrman's Nutritarian lifestyle is a powerful philosophy focused on health through a nutrient-rich, plant-based diet. The key principles really spoke to me:

Nutrient Density: Focus on foods that pack the most nutrients per calorie—like colourful vegetables, fresh fruits, hearty beans, healthy nuts, and whole grains.

Disease Prevention: Make choices that not only help prevent but can actually reverse chronic diseases like heart disease and diabetes.

Plant-Based Focus: Choose a mainly plant-based diet, limiting animal products and processed foods.

G-BOMBS: Emphasise the importance of nutrient-rich foods: Greens, Beans, Onions, Mushrooms, Berries, and Seeds.

Holistic Lifestyle: Include movement, stress management, and good sleep habits in your daily life.

Mindful Eating: Be aware of your food choices, fostering a loving relationship with what you eat.

Simplicity and Sustainability: Appreciate simple, home-cooked meals made with fresh ingredients, deepening your connection to health.

At its core, the Nutritarian philosophy gives hope, showing that what we eat can have a big impact on our health, longevity, and overall life quality. It empowers people to make smart choices that lead to better health and a stronger sense of well-being.

In that moment of inspiration and clarity, surrounded by warmth and friendship, I immediately signed up for Dr. Fuhrman's online membership and ordered his book *Eat to Live.*

Over the Christmas holiday, I lost myself in Dr. Fuhrman's book *Eat to Live* and his online materials, captivated by his clear and engaging teaching style. His lessons were a revelation, packed with helpful notes and extra resources that deepened my understanding. As I absorbed this knowledge, I had a powerful realisation: food is more than just fuel; it's an important act of self-care. What I chose to eat was a reflection of how I felt about myself. Choosing nourishing foods felt like showing myself love while ignoring my dietary needs felt like denying my worth.

This realisation hit me hard, connecting my growing understanding of self-compassion with my relationship with food for the first time. I felt ready to begin a transformative journey, one that would help me explore my true self. It was as if the universe had lined things up perfectly, offering me the clarity I needed at a turning point in my life. This guidance was leading me to a new phase of self-discovery, teaching me to deepen my ongoing journey of learning to love myself.

As I write this chapter of my book in mid-October 2024, I reflect on the significant milestones I've achieved. I've lost 25 kilograms since January 2024, reaching the size I was before having my twins – a size small. The confidence and self-love I've gained along with my physical transformation have been incredibly rewarding. Naturally, I needed an entirely new wardrobe, and this time, I chose bright colours and styles that celebrate the shape of my body—shapes I now embrace with pride. My renewed love for cooking has brought back fond memories of my childhood and my connection to food, making my journey even more meaningful.

My relationship with food has changed a lot over time. At first, I saw food only as a way to comfort myself and enjoy life, often turning to it when I was stressed or feeling emotional. This led to a cycle where I depended on food to feel better, but it often hurt my well-being. Food became a way to escape rather than something to nourish me.

But as I started to heal and understand myself better, I began to see food for what it really is: a way to take care of myself and a key part of being healthy. I learned to appreciate the value in the food I ate, realising that every meal is a chance to respect my body and mind. This shift in how I thought about food helped me build a healthier relationship with it, based on respect and gratitude, not just eating for the sake of it. Now, I approach food with intention. I choose foods that nourish my body and help me feel good. Eating has become a way of showing myself love. Each meal is a time for me to care for myself by choosing foods that boost my health and energy.

As I nurture this relationship, I've noticed how my love for myself has spread to other parts of my life. Eating well has improved my physical health, giving me more energy and mental clarity. It's also made me emotionally stronger, helping me face challenges with more positivity. The way I think about food now has also helped me connect more with who I am. Every meal is a celebration of my journey and a reflection of my values. I'm more aware of the tastes, textures, and origins of the food I eat, and this awareness has made me appreciate the variety and richness of food even more.

In the end, my acceptance of food's power isn't just about choosing what to eat; it's a deeper understanding of life itself. It reminds me that taking care of my body is a powerful act of self-compassion, and it affects all areas of my life. By honouring my relationship with food, I'm also honouring myself, creating a greater sense of fulfilment, joy, and connection to the world around me. The lessons I've learned through food have also helped me heal from childhood wounds that once held me back for years. Now, as I begin this new chapter, I feel like the timing is right—after working so hard on my mental and spiritual health, I'm finally giving my body the nourishment it needs. This journey of self-compassion, acceptance, and love isn't just about changing; it's about accepting who I am, celebrating my past, and moving forward into the future.

In Conclusion

As we reach the end of this chapter, I hope you've felt the essence of what I've tried to share. Each part of my story comes together to show the complexity of love in four key relationships:

1. Love as a Partner: Embracing the Journey of Marriage
2. Love as a Mother: Nurturing Bonds and Unconditional Connection
3. Love Among Family and Friends: The Strength of Cherished Connections
4. Nourishing Love: Cultivating a Relationship with What I Feed My Body

These relationships have not only made my life richer but have also taught me important lessons about connection, strength, and the power of love.

Through my stories, I've tried to show how love can lift us up and challenge us at the same time. Each relationship I've shared is like a chapter in my life filled with joy, heartache, and lessons that have shaped my understanding of what it really means to connect with others. The experiences I've had with family and friends have shown me how much we can learn from one another, each person adding something unique and meaningful to our lives.

In addition to these relationships, I've also shared my own journey of self-care, which has become so important to me. By focusing on my well-being and seeing nutrition as a form of self-love, I've learned how to nourish not only my body but my soul as well. This practice has helped me become more aware of myself and more compassionate, which has allowed me to give and receive love in a pure way. It's a reminder that the love we give others is often a reflection of the love we have for ourselves.

As I went deeper into the idea of love, I realised its paradox—the way it can both lift us up and challenge us at our core. I've thought about how my view of love has changed over the years, from something that caused me anxiety to something that gives me strength. This journey has taken me from holding onto love out of fear to embracing it as something empowering. It has allowed me to open my heart and share the love I was always meant to give.

Sarah Prout perfectly captures this journey in her book "Be the Love," saying, "When you learn to love yourself, you unlock the door to the greatest love of all—the love that flows effortlessly, freely, and abundantly." This quote deeply resonates with me, and it guides me as I continue to navigate the complexities of attachment and acceptance. It reminds me that real love starts within; by taking care of my heart, I've learned how to love others in a more genuine and complete way.

I hope that as you read my story, you found moments to think about your own experiences with love—the joys, the challenges, and the lessons that have shaped who you are. I trust you've seen that embracing love's dual nature can lead to a more fulfilling life, where we don't just love, but become love itself. My hope is that my journey inspires you to follow your own path of love, to appreciate the beauty in being vulnerable, and to value the relationships that make your life better. May you find something in my story that speaks to you and leaves you feeling empowered, ready to embrace the love you were always meant to share.

Spiritual Healing: Releasing the Wounds of the Past

In shadows deep, where sorrows hide,

A journey calls from far inside.

Where conscious thoughts and dreams collide,

To free the soul where pains reside.

The mind, a labyrinth worn by years,

Echoes softly, laced with fears.

But deep within, a whisper clears,

The light of truth, dissolving tears.

Through ancient wounds, the heart must tread,

To face the ghosts of what's unsaid.

The conscious and subconscious thread,

As one, they weave where you were led.

Old wounds stir, yet lose their reign,

Their chains dissolve in gentle rain.

With every step, the weight, the strain,

Unwinds and leaves a softer plane.

The self you buried, now reborn,

Emerges from the night forlorn.

Through healing's fire, the soul is worn,

And pain, once heavy, is outworn.

Now stand, with breath anew, set free,

The past is left beneath the tree

Of life, you climb, with unity,

The mind and soul are in harmony.

From depths, you rise, no more in flight,

With open wings, you seek the light.

Whole, complete, your soul shines bright,

In peace, you rest in truth's pure sight.

Introduction

As I set pen to paper, I reflect on the essence of my journey—a heartfelt odyssey through the shadows of my past, seeking the illuminating light of truth. For nearly four transformative years, I have explored the complexity of my mind and thoughts, daring to confront the fears and wounds that lingered like whispered echoes in the dark. This journey has been about more than mere self-discovery; it has been a tender reclamation of my identity, expanding from the roles that once defined me: as an executive, a wife, a mother, and a sister.

In this moment of reflection, I feel a deep resonance with lines that speak to ancient wounds and unspoken ghosts. The decision to part ways after a 19-year marriage was a heart-wrenching yet necessary step on my path to healing. The man I once loved, with all his admirable qualities, inadvertently triggered the cycles of familial pain I had sworn to break. This path required me to face those painful truths, echoing the poem's theme of confronting our shadows to find clarity and peace.

The imagery of chains dissolving in gentle rain beautifully captures my experience of shedding the weight of a high-powered job that no longer aligns with my true self. Leaving the corporate world felt like shedding a heavy cloak, granting me the freedom to explore the essence of who I am. I was no longer defined by titles or accolades but by the authenticity that lay within.

As a mother, I realised that to guide my twin boys towards living their own truths, I had to embody that truth myself. I endeavoured to demonstrate through my choices that genuine purpose arises from aligning with the deepest truths of our souls. This mirrors the poem's message of unity between the conscious and subconscious, where heart and mind balance harmoniously.

Yet, my journey also illuminated the neglect of my own body, often harmed by choices that failed to honour its needs. Embracing a Nutritarian lifestyle became a commitment and a sacred vow—a choice for vitality that echoed the poem's themes of renewal and rebirth.

Healing, however, demanded more than surface-level changes. While coaching and therapy provided a sturdy foundation, true transformation unfolded at a deeper, cellular level, as the poem so emotionally describes. This process could not be hurried; it blossomed in its own time, revealing layers of buried pain and allowing me to emerge stronger.

In this chapter, I wish to share two pivotal moments that catalysed profound spiritual healing—experiences that dissolved the barriers between my conscious and subconscious mind. These moments felt like revelations, yet they were more profound than mere experiences; they brought forth the freedom I had long sought, allowing me to reclaim my true self and step into the most authentic version of me. In the following weeks, I made decisions that sprang from intuition rather than logic, as if an energetic force was propelling me forward.

This chapter not only narrates my journey of deepening spiritual healing through two powerful experiences but also invites you, dear reader, to embrace your own journey through the shadows. May you recognise that every moment holds the potential for profound transformation, and may my story inspire you to seek your own light amidst the darkness.

Life Gives You What You Need and When You Need It

Life has a peculiar way of presenting us with exactly what we need, precisely when we need it. This thought often resonates within me, particularly when I reflect on the insights of Eckhart Tolle, who eloquently describes how life unfolds under the guidance of a higher intelligence. He reminds us that it is our responsibility to remain present and open to the opportunities that arise around us. When we fully embrace each moment, we tap into the vibrancy of the universe and the wisdom that flows through it. Tolle's poignant assertion that "life will give you whatever experience is most helpful for the evolution of your consciousness" strikes a deep chord within me. Each moment and every experience is a precious opportunity for spiritual growth and discovery.

Looking back on my own journey, I can see how life presented opportunities just when I needed them most. It took time for me to recognise my own readiness to receive them. My trip to the Amazon stands out as nothing short of incredible, arriving at a pivotal moment when I had stepped away from the relentless pace of the corporate world. I grappled with a nagging question that had become my constant companion: "Who am I?" This query haunted my thoughts daily, casting a shadow over my mind. Despite devouring nearly all of Michael Singer's works in search of answers, I found myself at a standstill, unable to respond.

Travelling with eleven wonderful people—fellow Board Members and Allies of the Foundation we supported—into the heart of the Amazon was a heartfelt privilege. As we journeyed deeper into the breathtaking rainforest, I felt a thrilling anticipation mingled with an anxiety of the uncertain. For ten months prior, I had engaged in a constant struggle to clear the overwhelming clutter from my mind, yearning to live each moment in harmony with the rhythm of life. The unending buzz of thoughts, worries, and distractions had left me feeling disconnected from the world around me. Ultimately, it was those transformative ten days spent immersed in the Amazon, alongside the Sàpara and Achuar communities, that allowed me to reach that long-awaited point of clarity.

Living in the jungle alongside the indigenous community, I found myself connecting with the essence of life in ways I had never imagined. Their wisdom and simple way of living opened my eyes to perspectives I'd never considered before. Their deep respect for every living thing and their ability to fully embrace the present moment touched me profoundly. During that time, I was forced to confront my fears. The unease I felt around the creatures scurrying about and my wariness of the murky jungle waters became challenges I was determined to face. Walking through the dense undergrowth on long treks pushed me to be brave, and floating down the river to return to camp became a soothing ritual for my spirit. For someone who had a deep fear of water and didn't know how to swim, floating down that river without fear felt like a miracle. I couldn't fully explain where this new confidence came from—it defied logic.

But it wasn't just the natural beauty that transformed me. The community's rituals and traditions brought about profound realisations. During these sacred moments, I started to peel away the layers of fear and doubt that had clouded my life. I began to see how many of my fears were shaped by my own perceptions and misconceptions. Taking part in their ceremonies, listening to their stories, and sharing in their laughter helped me uncover those layers, revealing truths about myself that I had long buried.

This journey gave me clarity about what it means to live with purpose while staying true to my values. When I returned home, my mind felt calm and still, free of the uncertainties that had weighed me down. I carried with me a new sense of excitement for life and the choices ahead. It was empowering, as though I'd been given the tools to shape my own destiny.

I will forever be grateful to the people of the Ecuadorian Amazon for welcoming us so openly and sharing their ancient wisdom. Their generosity and willingness to share their lives gave me the strength to overcome obstacles I hadn't even fully recognised before. Every smile and every shared connection reminded me that we are all part of something greater, a vast and interconnected web of life.

As Manari Ushigua said so beautifully, "I am taking you to the past (the forest), so that you can find solutions for the problems of the future (our modern world)." Those words resonate deeply with me. In that lush and vibrant jungle, I found answers to my questions and rediscovered a sense of purpose and belonging. Life, unpredictable as it is, keeps teaching me that when we open ourselves to its possibilities, we often find ourselves exactly where we need to be.

First Spiritual Healing Experience: Ayahuasca in the Ecuadorian Amazon Rainforest

As I sit down to share my first encounter with Ayahuasca, I invite you to journey with me into a world that is both mystical and deeply personal. This experience, rooted in the heart of the Ecuadorian Amazon, was not merely a rite of passage; it was a deep spiritual awakening, a dance with the essence of life itself. Guided by the esteemed Manari Ushigua, a Political and Spiritual Leader of the Sàpara people, I was enveloped in a ritual that transcended the ordinary, leading me into the depths of healing, self-discovery, and pure communion with the natural and spiritual realms.

The ceremony unfolded beneath the enchanting cloak of night within a traditional ceremonial hut where the vibrant sounds of the jungle formed a living backdrop to our intentions. Manari, with his deep-rooted wisdom and gentle presence, initiated our gathering with rituals that invited ancestral spirits to guide us. We prepared ourselves, both physically and mentally, through fasting and reflection, allowing the sacred plant medicine to cleanse our energies and open our hearts. As the sun dipped below the horizon, casting a golden glow that danced through the trees, a mixture of anticipation and nervousness swirled within me. The air was thick with the earthy scent of the Amazon, a reminder of the profound journey ahead. I carefully chose my yoga mat, crafting a small sanctuary amidst the vastness of the night, wrapped in a blanket of comfort and safety. My intention was clear yet heavy: to peel back the layers that had long obscured my true self, buried beneath years of expectations and obligations.

When the moment arrived, I watched others bravely step forward, each sipping the plant medicine we were offered. Their vulnerability stirred something profound within me, a sense of shared courage. Finally, it was my turn. Heart pounding, I approached the cup, drinking deeply, embracing the unknown ahead.

With my eyes closed, I whispered my question into the universe: "Who am I? Who am I?" This simple inquiry echoed through my mind, resonating with an urgency that felt both familiar and foreign. Time melted away as visions began to unfold—a kaleidoscope of shapes and colours pulsating against the dark canvas of my closed eyelids. Among them, I caught a glimpse of a woman moving gracefully, her silhouette unmistakably reminiscent of my mother, who had passed away years before. At that moment, confusion mixed with recognition, and my heart raced with the bittersweet feeling of her presence. I wanted answers, but they felt just out of reach. As I gave in to the experience, I was offered more Ayahuasca. I drank again, ready to explore this extraordinary journey further.

Then, as if something buried deep inside me was being stirred, a wave of nausea hit me hard. I called out for help, feeling vulnerable in both body and spirit. Someone guided me to the edge of the platform, and I leaned over, desperate to release everything building up inside me. In that moment of surrender, I felt it—a warm, steady hand on my back. Then, I heard my mother's voice, soft and comforting, saying, "It's okay. Let it out." With her gentle reassurance, the floodgates opened. I cried into the night, letting out everything I had been holding onto for so long. Each cry carried the truth of her love and reminded me that I was safe and cared for. "You are loved," she said again and again, wrapping me in a sense of connection that went beyond time and space.

When the purging finally stopped, I was helped back to my mat, feeling like a new person. The world around me seemed to glow with a dreamlike quality, as if everything had shifted. This journey with Ayahuasca wasn't just about personal healing; it was about connecting with ancient wisdom and understanding the deep ties that bind us all. It showed me the power of being vulnerable, of compassion, and of the unconditional love that flows through life, reminding us to embrace who we truly are.

Reflection on My Ayahuasca Experience

As I sit quietly and reflect on that life-changing morning, a wave of emotions washes over me, enveloping me in a tender embrace of nostalgia and revelation. The ceremony on the elevated platform felt like stepping into another realm—a sacred space where vulnerability was not just welcomed but celebrated. Sharing our stories was akin to peeling away the protective layers we so often wear, exposing the fragile parts of ourselves that long for understanding.

I still remember the astonishment I felt when I realised how much time had slipped away during my Ayahuasca journey. Hours had passed, yet it felt like only moments. Those moments, however, were packed with revelations that stayed with me long after. I was taken back to my earliest days as a baby—a time I couldn't consciously remember, but that had shaped the core of who I am. I saw myself, alone in a cot, crying for attention. The weight of that realisation hit me like a tidal wave. It wasn't just a memory but a direct encounter with the loneliness that had followed me through life.

Manari's words about encountering a spirit from my past suddenly made sense. That spirit turned out to be my mother—a woman who had faced her own struggles while raising ten children. As I reflected, I began to see the sacrifices she made, the strength of her faith, and the love she showed in her own imperfect way. I also became aware of the unspoken anger I had carried toward her, anger rooted in feelings of neglect and loneliness from my childhood. But as I looked deeper, I began to understand the truth: she had done the best she could, just as I try to do for my own children. In the calm of the Amazon, surrounded by the sounds of nature, I felt an overwhelming need to forgive—not just my mother, but myself too. I needed to forgive that little baby who felt unloved, who cried for connection, and whose pain later turned into anger. That part of me needed to be acknowledged and embraced with love.

My Ayahuasca journey wasn't just about revisiting the past. It was about learning to love myself, letting go of the hurt I had been holding onto, and finding a path to healing that I didn't know I needed. As those feelings ebbed and flowed, I felt a heavy burden lift from my shoulders. I realised the importance of showing that same love to my twin boys. The tenderness I felt for them blossomed and deepened. I could hold them not just physically but with my entire heart. Loving them transformed from duty into a joyful expression of the healing I had undergone.

Emerging from that experience felt like stepping into a new dawn. For the first time in years, I slept soundly, free from the insomnia that had plagued me. The wild beauty of the Amazon became a living symbol of my fresh beginning. I learned that tending to my own needs was not an act of selfishness; it was a vital necessity. I began to allow myself to feel emotions openly and to honour who I truly was.

Back in my corporate role, I felt a shift within me. I no longer sought validation from my title or achievements. I started to see myself simply as Rochelle—a leader, a mother, and a person deserving of love and respect. I granted myself permission to prioritise my health, future, and happiness.

As I continue to move forward, I carry with me the invaluable lessons I've learned—the love my mother expressed in her own way and the understanding that I am worthy of compassion. I'm learning to embrace my whole self and to nurture that child within me who once felt so utterly alone. In doing so, I am gradually uncovering the essence of who I truly am—someone deserving of love and capable of giving it freely.

Second Spiritual Healing Experience: Meditation Leveraging Modern Technology

I received an invitation to a meditation retreat that promised innovative methods for healing and personal growth—tools I felt were particularly relevant in today's challenging climate. When Dan mentioned Dr. Arne Heissel, the workshop leader, my curiosity was instantly piqued. Dr. Heissel, a former corporate leader turned modern mystic, energy healer, and visionary in global health, embodied a captivating blend of experience and insight that drew me like a moth to a flame. Having lived most of my life rationally and logically, I had always found solace in data and the transformative power of technology. I was eager to see how this modern approach could enhance my understanding of meditation.

Looking back, it's striking how perfectly everything fell into place. Meeting Dan and receiving that invitation felt like gifts from the universe, arriving precisely when I needed them most. At the time, I couldn't fully grasp the profound impact these experiences would have on my life, but a gentle voice within me urged, "Open your heart and let it unfold."

As I prepared for the retreat, a delightful blend of excitement and apprehension coursed through me. The idea of merging technology with meditation seemed revolutionary, and I was intrigued by how these seemingly disparate worlds could intersect. Would this experience challenge my logical mindset, or offer a new lens through which to view my reality?

Saturday morning dawned bright and clear, and I entered the retreat space, filled with excitement. The moment I stepped inside, a wave of energy washed over me, heightening my anticipation for the journey ahead. The room buzzed with connection as we gathered for our first session, each of us sharing our stories and the paths that had led us here. Hearing everyone's journeys made me feel united with them, weaving our individual tales into a rich tapestry of shared experience.

Our facilitator, Arne, spoke with a calm yet energising presence, outlining the journey we were about to embark upon. He highlighted its significance in today's hectic and troubled world, and as he spoke, a spark of hope ignited within me for the transformation that lay ahead. When Arne mentioned the subconscious mind, it struck a deep chord within me. He explained how it holds our beliefs and instincts, and how a non-purified subconscious mind may lead to a fear based stressed living, and an illusion of being in control, while a purified subconscious mind allows our brilliant mind to be in charge and allowing connection to a greater whole . This idea resonated, reminding me of the emotions and memories stored within me, often shaping my daily life while I ran on autopilot. It filled me with awe, and this moment offered me an opportunity to continue the journey I had begun years ago, striving to break free from old habits.

My curiosity intensified as Arne introduced the concept of measuring brain waves during meditation to assess different stages of consciousness. He elaborated on how scientists and himself use the state-of-the-art Vilistus Mind Mirror EEG technology to observe and train different brain wave patterns, each reflecting different states of awareness and creativity. In an ideal state, the Awakened Mind State, these waves harmonise, promoting a healthy mental flow state as our new ordinary state, which also serves as a springboard in extraordinary states of consciousness, allowing metaphysical states and deep insights. The thought of EEG feedback helping individuals recognise and adjust their brain wave patterns was both fascinating and reassuring, hinting at deeper emotional clarity and self-awareness.

Eagerly, we settled into our seats, ready to embark on this journey of self-discovery. It was time to try out the EEG machine, an intriguing device designed to measure brain activity during meditation. As the electrodes were placed on my head, I marvelled at the advancements in technology, a far cry from the bulky machines of the past, seamlessly connecting to a laptop that would display our brain activity. While connected to the EEG machines, I participated in short meditations that opened new pathways of introspection and self-discovery.

In our first session, a sensualisation-focused meditation, I felt a mix of curiosity and scepticism. At first, focusing on colours was overwhelming—I struggled to visualise anything. But as I shifted my attention to my breath, the world around me seemed to come alive. I became keenly aware of the subtle hum of sounds, the sweetness of imagined scents, and the vivid sensations of picturing an aeroplane taking off. This practice taught me to fully engage with my senses, showing me how they could ground my meditation and deepen my self-awareness. I left the session feeling validated and intrigued, excited to see how tuning into my dominant senses could shape future meditations.

In the second meditation, as we were guided into an alpha /theta state and asked to become an animal. My subconscious instinctively decided to embody my British Shorthair cat, Lena. I was drawn to her calm and steady energy. As I imagined myself as her, I found joy in the simplicity of her world—playful, loving, yet assertive. Reflecting on her qualities made me realise the warmth and gentleness I wanted to bring into my own life. This stood in stark contrast to a previous meditation where I had visualised myself as a tiger, representing raw strength and resilience. Comparing the two experiences made me see how my inner needs had shifted. I was no longer searching for sheer power but instead craved connection and adaptability. These meditative experiences illuminated the traits I wished to nurture: Lena's affection and grace, alongside the tiger's strength. From Lena, I sought to retain her warmth and loving nature, reminding me of the importance of connection and gentleness in my interactions

Insights Gained from the Experience of Meditation with Sound Medicine

As the meditation retreat unfolded, I stepped into the enchanting world of sound medicine for the first time. Arne, our guide, introduced us to this captivating concept, and I felt an immediate spark of intrigue. Having studied under Dr. Jeffrey Thompson, a pioneer in sound healing, Arne shared how specific frequencies can aid healing and restore balance in our lives. Listening to his explanations of techniques like binaural beats and solfeggio frequencies, a sense of excitement bubbled within me. For most of my life, I had been more comfortable with hard evidence and data, so the idea that sound and voice could shift our minds into various states of consciousness — enhancing our mental and physical well-being—felt nothing short of a revelation. It was as if I had stumbled upon a hidden treasure, one that promised to unlock new parts of myself.

For the remainder of the retreat, we engaged in four extended meditations, each one a unique journey. Two sessions, in particular, linger in my memory, and I feel compelled to share the insights I gained from them.

One session resonated deeply with me, revealing how even in a profound meditative state, our minds can cling to the familiar, resisting change. This became especially poignant as I navigated the landscapes of my thoughts during meditation. The session began with a gentle guided journey, and I envisioned a cherished place. In my mind, I found myself atop a serene mountaintop, surrounded by endless green trees. The cool, fresh air filled my lungs, and the crackle of a campfire nearby created a comforting atmosphere. It was a sanctuary, an escape from life's relentless busyness—a moment where I clung desperately to the comfort of the past.

As we were led to enter a house, I imagined a large glass structure shimmering in the sunlight. Upon stepping inside, I was greeted by a hallway lined with mirrors. Smiling at my reflection, I felt enveloped in warmth and contentment. Yet, as I ventured deeper, darkness crept in, leading me to a black door that felt ominous and out of place. Even in this serene setting, I could sense my mind resisting the change that awaited me beyond that door.

When I opened it, I stepped into a stark room, where a shadowy figure hunched in the corner. Instantly, a sharp ache pierced my chest—a manifestation of the pain I had long been hesitant to face. Our guide encouraged us to think about how we might change the space, but I felt paralysed, unwilling to confront the heaviness of that moment. Instead, I fled back into the light, seeking refuge in a lilac-coloured room bursting with floral scents and brightness. I told myself that this room was perfect as it was, resisting the change that would come from revisiting the darker space.

When the meditation concluded, I felt groggy, as if emerging from a vivid dream. I shared my experience with the group, describing the unsettling figure and the complex emotions it stirred within me. Arne noticed my hesitation and gently encouraged me to return to those rooms with my eyes closed. As I was guided back, something shifted inside me. Tears streamed down my face as I confronted feelings I had suppressed for years. In that dark room, the shadow took a clearer shape—it was my ex-husband, embodying the pain I had carried from our relationship. I realised I had been clinging to the responsibility for his healing, a burden that was never mine to bear. In contrast, the floral room symbolised my children—the light and joy in my life. This moment of clarity was a powerful insight. When I shared this breakthrough with the group, their support was overwhelming. Despite knowing them for only a short time, they made me feel seen and understood. Their reflections helped me confront a truth I had long avoided: I had spent years hoping for a miraculous change in my ex-husband while neglecting my own needs and self-worth.

In the days that followed, I reflected deeply on the revelations the meditation had uncovered. I began to understand how my past shaped my ideas about love, intertwining it with sacrifice and service. My efforts to prove my worth had left scars that influenced my relationships and choices. I recognised that both my ex-husband and I were struggling with our own wounds, unable to provide the love we needed to each other. Our marriage had become a cycle of hurt rooted in our unresolved pasts. While I treasure the memories we shared and the beautiful sons we raised, I now see that true healing requires both individuals to be ready. I couldn't change him; he had to forge his own path. Acknowledging this truth brought a profound sense of gratitude for the lessons I've learned. I feel thankful for the love and pain that shaped who I am today.

This meditation served as yet another turning point in my journey. It reminded me of the importance of self-love and the necessity of breaking free from patterns that no longer serve me. With love and respect for my past, I know I need to move forward into a brighter chapter, embracing the light while accepting the shadows. This experience wasn't just an exploration of my subconscious—it was a pivotal moment in my ongoing journey of healing and self-discovery, allowing me to let go of clinging and embrace the transformative power of change.

Another meditation session that particularly resonated with me was my journey to reconnect with my inner child. During my Ayahuasca experience in the Amazon, I encountered profound emotions that transported me back to the age of two, where I felt a powerful connection with my mother's spirit. This brought immense healing, yet during this meditation, it became clear that there was still more to address from my childhood. It underscored the non-linear nature of healing; various experiences can illuminate different aspects of our past. From the very beginning, Arne's soothing voice transported me to a sacred space. His gentle words enveloped me, drawing me into the experience as if I were not merely listening but fully immersed. It felt deeply personal, inviting me to reflect on my life and embark on an inward journey.

As the meditation progressed, I began to feel cold. Soon, vivid images from my childhood emerged—not random but clear scenes that played out like a film of my life, each moment imbued with emotion. This return to my inner child perfectly aligned with the session's intention. When Arne invited us to express gratitude for our inner child, an overwhelming wave of emotion washed over me. My body, once cold, began to warm, particularly around my heart. Tears streamed down my face—tears of joy and love—as I honoured my younger self, recognising her courage and showering her with the love she had always deserved. Then, unexpectedly, my body began to shake lightly, starting with small tremors in my legs. The shaking moved upwards, alternating between each leg and then to my chest. I was acutely aware of these sensations, and despite still feeling cold, I was amazed by the experience unfolding within me. When the meditation concluded, I struggled to recall how I had been guided back. I found myself sitting up, holding my head, attempting to process the depth of what I had just experienced. I felt physically exhausted and a tightness in my forehead, but also profoundly moved.

Later, Arne confirmed that my body had indeed been shaking. He explained that this response is natural, similar to how animals release tension after wounds. It was my body's way of letting go of stored pain and negative energy buried deep within my subconscious. I was astonished that sound and high gamma frequencies could elicit such a powerful physical and emotional release. It reminded me of a similar experience during an Ayahuasca ceremony in the Amazon, where I also encountered body tremors. I had never considered that sound alone could provoke such profound effects.

Reflecting on these moments, I realised that each meditation had peeled away layers I hadn't even known were there. They unearthed the forgotten fragments of my childhood, allowing me to embrace the innocence and vulnerability of my younger self. This connection was a reminder that healing is not a straight path; it is a winding journey that reveals itself unexpectedly.

As I continue on this path of self-discovery, I carry with me the lessons learned from both the dark corners of my psyche and the radiant light of my inner child. Each experience has taught me that true healing involves honouring all parts of myself—the joyous and the painful. It is in this balance that I find strength and resilience. With a renewed sense of purpose, I am committed to nurturing my inner child and embracing the wonder and curiosity that come with it. I am learning to create a safe space within myself, where I can explore my emotions without fear or judgement. This journey of self-love is ongoing, but with each step, I feel more empowered to rewrite my narrative, weaving together the threads of my past into a tapestry of hope and healing. In essence, these meditations have opened doors to a deeper understanding of who I am and who I aspire to be. They have illuminated the path ahead, reminding me that while the shadows may linger, the light of self-compassion and love shines ever brighter. And so, I move forward, heart open and ready to embrace the beautiful complexities of my journey.

In the days that followed my retreat, I found myself enveloped in a warm cocoon of reflection. The experience had been profound, and as I delved into why animals shake after moments of fear, a deeper understanding blossomed within me. I learned that this trembling is nature's way of helping them release pent-up tension and reset their nervous systems. It struck me then how similar we are as humans; we, too, carry wounds, often nestled deep within our bodies, waiting for a moment to be acknowledged and released.

Over the years, my journey through therapy had been focused on managing my triggers and developing coping strategies. Yet, I had often skirted around the root causes of my wounds, not fully confronting the wounds that lay beneath the surface. This meditation served as a gentle nudge, encouraging me to face those deep-seated hurts. It resonated with my Ayahuasca experience, where I had bravely confronted childhood wounds and unshackled long-held anger. In this meditation, I revisited various moments from my early years, gaining fresh perspectives on the insecurities they had instilled in me.

One memory that vividly emerged was of me, at the tender age of five, guiltily sipping from my niece's baby bottle. It was a small, innocent act, yet it revealed a profound longing for attention—a need that had manifested in ways I hadn't fully understood, leaving emotional scars in its wake. Another recollection was of a teacher who once told me I'd never amount to anything, due to my rebellious spirit and frequent mischief. Those words clung to me for years, igniting a relentless drive to succeed and prove my worth.

Despite having crafted a life that many would envy—a loving family, financial security, and a successful career—I often found myself grappling with a sense of unfulfillment. This meditation allowed me to sift through those formative moments, comprehend how they had shaped my identity, and release the pain they had imposed. It was a gentle reminder that I was never broken; I had always been a beautiful, whole child, deserving of love and acceptance. The tears that flowed during this session were cathartic, an acknowledgement of my journey and a loving embrace of my past. By reconnecting with my inner child, I released the pain that had taken residence deep within my body and subconscious. This transformative experience illuminated the joy and wholeness of the person I had always been at my core.

Eckhart Tolle, in his enlightening book *"The Power of Now",* speaks of the necessity of silencing the mind to access deeper spiritual awareness and presence. He suggests that much of our suffering springs from an overactive mind, and finding stillness is pivotal to achieving peace and awakening. This meditation brought that lesson to life in a way that was profoundly impactful for me. It served as a poignant reminder of the power of self-love and the importance of showing up authentically with one another, irrespective of our tumultuous pasts. This was a gentle reminder that healing isn't a singular event but rather a continuous journey. The trembling I experienced was my body's way of finding peace and releasing what no longer served me. This meditation experience echoed my previous Ayahuasca journey, reinforcing the idea that healing is not linear. Each experience—whether through meditation or other means—unveils new layers of understanding and growth. Ultimately, this meditation retreat was far more than a collection of sessions; it was a sacred reminder of the power of healing, the beauty of shared human connection, and the imperative of living from a place of love and acceptance.

In Conclusion

As I set out on a journey to discover my true self, I was fortunate to experience two life-changing paths. One led me deep into the Ecuadorian Amazon, guided by Manari Ushigua, a spiritual healer from the Sàpara Nation. The other took place in the peaceful surroundings of a meditation retreat in Switzerland, led by Dr. Arne Heissel, where ancient mindfulness practices blended seamlessly with modern technology. Both experiences were transformative, each offering unique insights into self-discovery.

The Ayahuasca ceremony with Manari felt like stepping into a vivid dream. The rainforest buzzed with life, wrapping me in its vibrant energy. Sitting in a circle with others searching for answers, I was surrounded by the earthy scent of damp soil and the sounds of the jungle at night. In that moment, I felt deeply connected to everything around me. Manari, calm and wise, began the ritual by calling on the spirits of plants and ancestors. When I drank the sacred Ayahuasca medicine, I did so with reverence, aware of its power to reveal truths I hadn't faced.

As the plant medicine coursed through me, I felt a profound connection to nature. It was as if the plants whispered their wisdom, the animals offered guidance, and the earth itself embraced me. I encountered the spirit of Ayahuasca, often represented as a serpent, which shared lessons about healing and purpose. The physical purging—vomiting and sweating—was more than a bodily release; it was an emotional and spiritual cleanse that helped me let go of old wounds. This wasn't just a personal healing experience; it was a bridge to the ancestral wisdom of the Sàpara people, helping me understand their way of life more deeply.

In contrast, the meditation retreat in Switzerland appealed to my rational and analytical side. Here, modern technology played a central role, and I was drawn to the precision of data and science. The retreat was structured and intentional, blending ancient practices with innovative tools. The calm, welcoming space introduced me to devices like EEG monitors that tracked brain activity. There was a sense of purpose in the air—a sanctuary for building resilience and awareness. Dr. Heissel, steady and encouraging, guided us through meditative exercises enhanced by sound therapy and breathwork.

These sessions took me on a different kind of journey. The rhythmic sounds and Dr. Heissel's gentle prompts helped me dive into states of consciousness I hadn't explored before. Unlike the raw, primal connection I felt during the Ayahuasca ceremony, this was an inward exploration focused on understanding the mind and body. The EEG readings offered real-time feedback, which appealed to my logical nature and reassured me about the process.

Though vastly different, both experiences shared a common goal: healing and self-discovery. The Ayahuasca ceremony taught me to surrender to the wisdom of nature and spirit, while the meditation retreat gave me tools to better navigate my inner world. Together, they showed me two sides of the same coin—one grounded in the earth and spirit, the other centred on the mind and modern innovation.

As these experiences came to an end, I carried their lessons with me. The Amazon journey reminded me of my connection to nature and the interconnectedness of life. The meditation retreat provided practical strategies to build resilience and find calm in a fast-paced world.

Both paths revealed the complexity of healing. The ancient wisdom of the Amazon and the structured mindfulness of Switzerland offered unique ways to explore my soul. They encouraged me to embrace both the wild, untamed beauty of nature and the quiet strength within myself. In this balance, I began to understand not only who I am but who I might become.

Looking back, I realise these experiences came at exactly the right time in my life. My meditation retreat felt richer because of my time in the Amazon. Each experience built on the other, showing me that life is a continuous journey of growth. I also learned how much I lean on logic, which can sometimes hold me back from flowing with life's unpredictability. While rational thinking is valuable, it's just as important to trust intuition and find inspiration in the natural world. Neither experience was better than the other; instead, they highlighted the value of different perspectives in guiding us forward.

As we conclude this chapter of exploration and insight, I invite you to pause and reflect on your own journey. Consider the moments that have shaped you—the experiences that have compelled you to confront your true self, whether through nature's wild embrace or the calm sanctuary of introspection. Embrace the duality of your path, recognising that both the chaotic and the serene play essential roles in your growth. Each journey, no matter how different, contributes to a richer understanding of who you are and aspire to be. Let the lessons of the earth and the mind intertwine within you, guiding you toward a deeper connection with yourself and the world around you. As you navigate your own exploration of self, remember that the beauty of life often lies in embracing the complexity of the journey itself.

FREEDOM FOUND: EMBRACING AUTHENTICITY

In South Africa's sunlit embrace,

A journey began, a quest to retrace,

Trading the mask for a life more true,

Manifesting dreams that once felt askew.

With courage ignited, they turned within,

Peeling back layers, where authenticity could begin,

Wounds of the past laid bare to the light,

Finding the strength to reclaim their might.

Books whispered wisdom, guiding the way,

Transformative tales of bold, vibrant sway,

Through wound's embrace, they learned to be whole,

Vulnerability's power, the key to the soul.

From corporate towers, they chose to depart,

Chasing authenticity, a leap from the heart,

In the Amazon's depths, they found their release,

Nature's calm cradle, a sanctuary of peace.

With pen and with silence, new practices bloomed,

Journalling thoughts, in stillness consumed,

Each moment a lesson, each breath a new chance,

Embracing the chaos, inviting the dance.

A life reimagined, values held dear,

Dreams nurtured gently, banishing fear,

Balancing passion and needs intertwined,

Manifesting a future, uniquely defined.

Relationships blossomed, like tides on the shore,

Prioritising joy, opening each door,

In honesty's light, true connections took flight,

Crafting a circle that felt just right.

Rochelle Trow

Curiosity sparked, the unknown now bright,

Embracing the journey, igniting the night,

With each step uncharted, new passions arose,

In the arms of uncertainty, the spirit grows.

Releasing the burden of control's tight embrace,

Finding peace in acceptance, discovering grace,

In stillness and presence, a sanctuary found,

Gratitude blossomed, joy's sweet sound.

Resilience emerged from the shadows of pain,

Transforming each setback, growth in the rain,

Every challenge a teacher, each trial a guide,

A tapestry woven with love deep inside.

Now, empowered to share, they step forth anew,

A beacon of light, inspiring the few,

Creating a legacy, compassionate and bold,

Inviting all seekers to let their dreams unfold.

In the heart of transformation, the journey is clear,

From longing to living, igniting sincere,

Each life holds a story, a chance to ignite,

A vibrant existence, embracing the light.

Beyond Myself: Discovering the Wholeness Within

In this book, I shared the stories that shaped me, starting with my upbringing in South Africa. Those early days were filled with innocence, curiosity, love, and joy. But as I grew older, I unknowingly built walls around my heart to protect myself, cutting off the richness of life in the process.

Looking back, I see how I changed from a bright-eyed child into someone I hardly recognised. In trying to feel safe, I shut down parts of myself. It felt like the right thing to do at the time, but it left me disconnected from who I really was. The constant noise in my head drowned out the world around me, leaving me feeling isolated and exhausted. Insomnia became a part of my life, and I often felt like I was spiralling out of control, trapped in a storm of chaotic thoughts. On the surface, I had everything I thought I wanted—financial security, a loving husband, children, a great job, and wonderful friends. But underneath, I felt painfully empty. I wore my achievements like a badge, but deep down, I was lost. I missed the curious child I used to be, the one who found comfort in books and imagined endless possibilities. Despite giving so much to those around me, I felt unloved, as though nothing came back in return.

Then everything fell apart, forcing me to take a hard look at myself—not in the mirror, but deep inside. It felt like peeling away layers of an onion, slowly breaking down the walls I had built around my heart. I remembered the teachings of Michael Singer, who spoke about the need for liberation, and Philip Shepherd's words in *Radical Wholeness*: "Reconnecting with the fullness of our being begins with the courage to dismantle the walls we've built." These words reminded me that it takes bravery to reclaim your authentic self. I began to ask myself, *Who am I, really?* In moments of quiet reflection, I realised my life often felt like a performance. The roles I played—mother, wife, sister, friend and executive —hid my true self. My heart said one thing, but my mind shouted another, and the conflict left me anxious and stifled.

As I explored this further, I realised this tension wasn't just an annoyance but a wake-up call. Something had to change. I needed to let go of the relentless mental chatter and embrace the freedom that came with being my true self. Letting go wasn't easy, but it was the only way to tear down the barriers keeping me from fully experiencing life. It marked the start of a journey back to the curious, vibrant child I once was and toward a life filled with love and authenticity.

Self-Reflection Leading to Growth

The journey of looking inward wasn't easy, but it was the most transformative experience of my life. It started with an urgent need to quiet the chaos in my mind and ease the heavy feeling in my chest. The constant churn of thoughts left me feeling trapped, pushing me to seek answers. I initially found comfort in books, shelves filled with wisdom and the hope of understanding. I devoured self-help books, desperate to make sense of my feelings and unravel the confusion that had me feeling so lost. My niece, Melanie, recommended books that became guiding lights along the way. Titles like *What Happened to You?* by Dr. Bruce Perry and Oprah Winfrey helped me understand how wounds shape us. *The Untethered Soul* by Michael Singer taught me the importance of inner peace, while Brené Brown's *Daring Greatly* showed me the power of vulnerability. Elizabeth Gilbert's *Eat, Pray, Love* mirrored my struggles with self-discovery, and Marisa Peers' *I Am Enough* reminded me of my worth. Each book offered insights, but I still felt like parts of the puzzle were missing.

Understanding my inner world through rational logic was just the first step. The real challenge was turning those insights into transformational change. Fear of the unknown held me back. I wonder*ed what would happen if I stepped outside my comfort zone.* One of my many breakthrough moments came during a coaching session with my coach. She helped me see the importance of staying true to my values and focusing on what really mattered to me. That realisation felt like a revelation—I didn't have to mould myself to fit a life that wasn't meant for me. With this clarity, I created a vision for freedom—the freedom to be myself. I pictured Nelson Mandela gazing into a sunset, his words ringing in my ears: "As we let our own lights shine, we unconsciously give others the permission to do the same." This quote became my mantra, guiding me as I began listing the values I wanted to live by. It quickly became apparent that major changes were needed in my life.

I began working on a four-year plan, a roadmap to a new life. The first step was addressing my marriage, a difficult but necessary decision. In the second year, I tackled my unhealthy relationship with work. By chance—or perhaps fate—an opportunity arose to leave my job, and I took it, determined to take time out from the corporate world to rediscover myself. Year three was all about growth and exploration. I took a parenting course and engaged in coaching sessions with my children, building stronger connections with them. I started meditating and journaling, searching for meaning in my experiences. A trip to the Amazon was a turning point, where spiritual healing ceremonies freed me from one of my most significant childhood scars and reawakened a sense of wonder within me. For the first time in years, I woke up without a rigid plan. I allowed myself to enjoy small moments, like a simple cup of coffee, and embraced the freedom to just *be.* It was uncomfortable at first but also the most liberating decision I had ever made. By year four, I turned my attention to my health. I wanted to shed the extra weight I had gained over the years, but this time, it wasn't just about appearances—I wanted to do it for the right reasons. A chance lunch with a close friend introduced me to Dr. Joel Fuhrman's nutritarian lifestyle. This approach became my guiding light for the year, helping me make meaningful changes aligned with the acceptance and growth I nurtured over the past three years.

Everything I had worked on—my marriage, career, identity, and health—was deeply connected. Each decision I made helped lay the foundation for the next, creating a path to success. The transformation wasn't just physical; it was also deeply personal. I rediscovered the vibrant, energetic woman I once was. Through this journey, I learned that true freedom comes from within. It's a steady light that remains even in the darkest moments. This path taught me compassion—not just for myself, but for the people around me. Inspired by Mandela's words, I now strive to be a light for others, sharing the lessons I've learned to help them on their journeys.

Reflecting on my Journey of Healing and Self-Discovery

For four long years, challenges seemed to follow me everywhere. No matter how carefully I planned or how big my dreams were, life had a way of throwing me off course, forcing me to confront fears I thought I had buried. My biggest struggle was learning to move out of my head and into my heart—a journey that sometimes felt endless.

Immersing myself in books was a natural action for a rational, logical me and a comfort zone to be surrounded by facts, trying to make sense of what I was reading. Still, I had to accept that I needed to do more, so I spent hours in therapy with psychologists and psychiatrists over the years, pouring out my emotions. But I soon realised I was only scratching the surface of my insecurities. Simply recognising old wounds and triggers wasn't enough to set me free. I kept asking myself, "How do I truly let go of this pain? How do I finally move past the weight of my childhood wounds?" The answers came slowly, through spiritual healing ceremonies and deep meditation that brought me closer to my inner child. Over those four years, I meditated for hours, trying to reframe the stories I had been telling myself about my past. I told that little girl inside me that the lessons she learned back then were flawed, based on beliefs that no longer served me. Still, the pain remained. It wasn't until I took part in powerful experiences, like ayahuasca healing ceremonies in the Amazon and sound and deep meditations using soundwaves, that I felt a real shift. These moments opened the floodgates, allowing me to release emotions and trapped pain I had been holding onto for years.

One day, a moment of pure inspiration changed everything. After spending eight months writing sporadically, I suddenly found myself filled with creativity. Over the course of just 16 days, I completed what I had struggled with for months. It all began after a meditation retreat. On the morning of October 7, 2024, I woke up at 4 AM with a clarity and energy I hadn't felt in years. Words started pouring out of me as if they had been waiting for this moment to be released. What started as a gift for my children turned into something much bigger: a way to share my story and connect with others who had experienced similar struggles. The meditation retreat enabled me to continue releasing wounds I had started to heal back in the Amazon, but it was now clear that I needed more healing. The retreat allowed me to release even more old wounds, which gave me the clarity to see my purpose—I knew this story needed to be told. In the weeks that followed, my writing process underwent a remarkable transformation. The chapters that had once felt insurmountable suddenly fell into place, as I reconnected with the creative parts of myself that had been dormant for so long.

I began each chapter by writing a poem to encapsulate the emotions and themes I wanted to explore. This process reminded me that triggers never truly vanish; they simply become more familiar and more manageable. As my familiar self-doubt crept in, whispering that my poems weren't good enough. My pursuit of perfection led me to seek support from AI, turning the process of polishing my verses into a collaborative, creative adventure. Once I had shaped my poems, I poured my thoughts into the recorder, my gaze continuously fixed on their stanzas as I spoke. Writing became a cathartic release, allowing me to unearth emotions I had bottled up for years. Some moments surprised me, particularly when my tone shifted while revisiting painful memories or reflecting on my ex-husband. I was compelled to confront my anger and fear, but as I pressed on, I discovered love and acceptance waiting patiently on the other side. Once the recordings were complete, I would sit down behind my Mac screen to refine the text, but the essence of those initial outpourings remained at the heart of my book.

Through this process, I learned to embrace all parts of myself, even the ones I had tried to ignore. I found new ways to cope with my past—ways that brought me joy and nourished my soul. By October 23, 2024, I had written the final chapter of my manuscript for the book. It was a testament to the transformative power of that serendipitous moment and the focus that followed.

Looking back, I now recognise that the end of my marriage was a significant hurdle during this period. Growing up in a family that held marriage in such high esteem, admitting that mine had failed felt like a heavy burden to bear. I had to confront my feelings of inadequacy and the expectations of others who viewed us as the perfect couple. Initially, I grappled with the label of 'failure,' but as I wrote, I came to realise that my journey was not about defeat. We were two imperfect individuals brought together by chance, each carrying our own emotional scars. These scars became even more pronounced as I struggled to accept his behaviour. I transitioned from deep anger that clouded my judgement to a rational understanding of what our situation meant. However, it wasn't until I truly let go of expecting anything in return that I could free myself from the marriage. This long, arduous, and painful process took nearly four years, and just today, as I make the final edits to this chapter, we are finally close to alignment on the divorce agreement. Understanding that our relationship wasn't meant to last didn't erase the invaluable lessons I learned during nearly two decades together. It became clear that we were better apart—not just for ourselves but also for our children. That realisation was liberating; it lifted the weight of societal expectations from my shoulders, allowing me to embrace a future filled with possibility.

Another challenge I faced was my career. As I climbed the corporate ladder, I felt proud of my accomplishments, but over time, I realised my motivation was misplaced. I didn't need a prestigious title; I wanted work that felt meaningful and aligned with my values. When I finally decided to step back from my career, I sensed my family's doubt and hesitation. This shift taught me a hard but valuable lesson about relationships. Many people I thought were friends drifted away when my title changed. At first, it hurt—it bruised my ego—but

I came to understand that those who valued me only for my job weren't true friends. I began to focus my energy on building deeper, more genuine connections. As I embraced authenticity, my circle of friends evolved. I started attracting people who shared my values and people who found purpose beyond job titles. The energy I put into the world changed, and in return, I found relationships that were rich with meaning and true connection.

Standing on the other side of these obstacles, with my book now complete, I can see how far I've come. I've learned that real freedom comes from within—accepting my journey, my pain, and my growth. In that acceptance, I've found a deep sense of peace and liberation. It's allowed me to fully embrace life, with all its beauty and challenges, as it unfolds. Every challenge I faced became a stepping stone, helping me understand myself and the world more deeply. I've come to see how all my experiences—whether heartbreaks, victories, or quiet moments of reflection—have woven together the story of my life. Whether joyful or painful, each moment has added depth and meaning to the story I now share with others.

As I built new relationships, I discovered the power of vulnerability. Opening up about my struggles allowed others to do the same, creating a safe space where we could connect on a deeper level. I realised that true connection grows when we're honest about who we are—flaws and all. Being open about my imperfections brought a sense of belonging I had longed for.

Writing my book has become more than just recounting my past—it's been a way to heal. The process of putting my emotions into words has helped me understand and honour my journey. Sharing my story also invites others to reflect on their own lives, accept their experiences, and find comfort in knowing they're not alone. With each chapter, I'm reclaiming my voice and creating a space for others to hear theirs. I hope my words reach people who feel lost, are wrestling with their struggles, and are looking for acceptance and understanding. By sharing my truth, I want to encourage others to start their own journeys of healing and self-discovery.

Embracing My Rebel Within

My journey took an incredible amount of courage—the kind that pushes you into the unknown and forces you to walk paths that most wouldn't dare to explore. It was scary, and it took months to make the decisions I eventually arrived at. I won't pretend the struggle wasn't real. Finding courage wasn't easy; it required me to dig deep, and face fears head-on. But in doing so, I uncovered my inner rebel. This time, though, my rebellion had a purpose. I stood up for what I believed in and embraced the truths that felt right for me. When I was younger, my rebellion came from a need to protect myself—it was my way of resisting anything that tried to crush my spirit. But now, I was rebelling out of love: love for myself, compassion for others, and the desire to accept myself fully. I realised that by caring for myself, I could become the person I was meant to be. It's like the advice they give on planes—put on your oxygen mask first before helping others. I needed to make my well-being a priority so I could show up fully for my children.

This meant examining the external pressures in my life and setting clearer boundaries in my relationships. I had to think carefully about who I let into my inner circle, who I shared my time and energy with, and what kind of vibes I allowed into my life. It wasn't about cutting people off but about being thoughtful and intentional about where I invested my energy. I've come to accept that not everyone in my life operates on the same wavelength, and that's okay. We're all on different journeys, and it's not appropriate for me to judge anyone else's path. But within my own life, I have the power to decide whose energy I want to keep close. I get to choose which connections uplift me and which ones, for my own sake, I need to let go of. This clarity gave me a sense of strength and resilience I hadn't felt before. For the first time, I felt confident in making decisions that aligned with who I truly was. I followed my own inner compass and finally tuned into what I needed and wanted.

Through this process, I realised that self-care isn't selfish—it's essential. By surrounding myself with positive, supportive energy, I could be more authentic. This didn't just benefit me; it allowed me to show up more fully for my children and the people I love. I started to appreciate the relationships that brought joy and growth into my life, while gently stepping away from those that drained me. This deliberate choice to protect my energy became an act of self-love. It was my way of saying I deserve to thrive in an environment that reflects my values and goals. I learned to listen to my intuition and trust the voice inside me that pointed me toward what felt right. As I did, I became more aware of my own needs and desires, letting my heart lead the way.

I began to see life as a constant exchange of energy. By aligning myself with positivity and purpose, I created an inner space where I could grow and flourish without fear of judgment or negativity. Choosing this path felt like a quiet rebellion against a world that often tells us who we should be and how we should live.

Through all this, I learned that strength isn't about never feeling afraid; it's about facing those fears with kindness and compassion. By standing up for myself, I found that I could also lift others up, creating an atmosphere where mutual support and encouragement could thrive. This cycle of giving and receiving became a cornerstone of my life, proving how powerful it can be to embrace your inner rebel. So I kept moving forward, taking the lessons I'd learned and the love I'd nurtured along the way. I welcomed every challenge, knowing it was another chance to grow and become more of the person I was meant to be. No longer just surviving, I was thriving—rooted in my truth and blossoming into the vibrant, authentic self I had always hoped to become.

As I write the final lines of this chapter, I feel deeply grateful. Every setback, every moment of doubt, and every glimpse of hope has brought me to this point. I feel stronger now, ready to move forward—not as someone defeated by life's challenges but as someone who has grown through them and is eager to face what's next. In this place of acceptance, I understand that my journey isn't over. Life will always bring challenges, but I'm no longer afraid of them. Every experience is a chance to grow and to understand love, connection, and purpose better. I'm ready to welcome whatever comes next, with an open heart and a willingness to embrace the beauty and complexity of life.

Embracing the Unknown: Welcoming Future Possibilities

In this chapter, I want to tie together the ideas and experiences I've shared throughout this book, creating a narrative that highlights my transformation. Reflecting on how I've learned to let go of control and embrace the unknown, I'll touch on key moments that shaped this mindset and opened new doors for me. Curiosity and exploration have been constant themes in my journey, and I'll focus on how these helped me discover new interests and passions. These explorations led to opportunities I hadn't expected, enriching my life and giving me a deeper understanding of myself and the world.

I'll also reflect on times when I stepped outside my comfort zone and took risks. These experiences taught me valuable lessons and changed how I see life. The emotions I felt during these moments—fear, excitement, and eventually, triumph—played a big role in shaping who I am today. As I look ahead, I'll share my aspirations and explain how they've been shaped by the lessons I've learned from embracing change. Together, we'll look at what it means to navigate uncertainty and how those insights can guide us moving forward. This chapter is the culmination of everything we've explored, a reminder of the power of letting go, staying curious, and accepting life's unpredictability. I hope it inspires you to see the unknown as a place full of possibilities waiting to unfold.

The Art of Letting Go

Letting go has been one of the most challenging lessons for me to learn. It felt like I was battling shadows in my own mind, constantly wrestling with an inner voice that wouldn't quiet down. Michael Singer captures this struggle perfectly—the relentless mental chatter that insists we must control everything. For a long time, I found solace in the belief that I could manage the chaos; I thought that if I clung tightly enough, I could dictate the outcomes in my life. Yet deep down, I knew this wasn't true. My need for control had become a snare. I was so fixated on the immediate—the dishes piling up, my children's schedules, the weight of expectations—that I overlooked the beauty surrounding me. Letting go meant changing a lot of habits. I had to let go of needing a spotless house, the urge to make my kids stick to rigid routines, and the expectation that they should always act perfectly polite, just like I was taught.

My desire for justice and fairness morphed into another form of control, draining my energy as I fought for fairness against someone who, truth be told, would never relinquish the sanctuary he had built around his own version of the truth. It became a battle of egos, both of us clinging to control, which ultimately left us trapped in a cycle. It wasn't until I chose to let go of my need for justice that I began to free myself. I realised it wasn't my responsibility to dictate the situation; the universe would address him in its own time. This prolonged struggle kept us legally separated, but not divorced for nearly four years.

One day, I decided to step back, at least in my mind. I imagined looking at my life from outer space. In that vast perspective, I saw myself as just a tiny speck—a grain of sand on an endless beach. It was humbling. It made me realise how small I was in the grand scheme of things. If I was just one tiny grain, how could I possibly think I could control everything?

This idea reminded me of Eckhart Tolle's teachings about living in the present. He talks about how the ego tricks us into thinking we need control, keeping us stuck in a cycle of dissatisfaction. True peace, he says, comes from letting go and being fully present in the moment. With this perspective, I realised that the only thing I could really control was myself—how I reacted, what I thought, and the energy I put into the world. Reaching an understanding of the need to let go wasn't easy. I made plenty of mistakes, particularly in the early years, as I grappled with the process. Fortunately, I stumbled upon practices that proved invaluable—mindfulness, journaling, meditation, and spending time in nature. These tools became my anchors in the storm of my thoughts. Tolle speaks about observing your thoughts without judgment, and I found that this practice created space for genuine change in my life.

Leaving the corporate world was a significant step for me. It granted me the time and space to slow down, calm my restless mind, and confront the endless list of "musts" and my obsession with justice and fairness. When I envisioned that beach filled with grains of sand, I realised just how unrealistic it was to believe I could control every single one of those things. Learning to quiet my mind, which incessantly chattered about everything I tried to control, felt like liberation.

One particularly memorable moment of calm occurred during a spiritual healing session in the Amazon rainforest. During that meditation, I experienced the profound sensation of a completely quiet mind and craved more of that stillness in my life. Nestled in the heart of the jungle, surrounded by the hum of insects and the rustling of leaves, I discovered a deep sense of peace. The Amazon became a sanctuary for me, vibrant with life yet filled with tranquillity. I began healing old wounds through spiritual ceremonies with the local communities. My mind quieted, and I felt an intimate connection with the world around me.

Now, I live with so much gratitude. I can appreciate the present moment without being weighed down by the past or worrying about the future. Life feels brighter and more open, and I notice people and experiences that had always been there but that I was too distracted to see. I feel more connected to others, and this connection fills me with love and joy.

Letting go has been one of the hardest battles of my life, but it's also been the most freeing. I wish I had learned to do it sooner. So many of us are trapped in the constant noise of our own minds, missing out on the beauty right in front of us. Letting go isn't just a choice; it's a way of freeing our souls, allowing us to live truly. As both Singer and Tolle have said, real freedom comes from surrendering control and embracing the present moment, letting life unfold as it's meant to.

Finding My Curiosity Again

There was a time when I felt like a puppet, my strings pulled tight by the endless demands of life. I was caught in a cycle of control, trying to manage every little thing, only to feel more lost with each passing day. It was during this overwhelming period that I learned one of life's most valuable lessons: how to let go. Slowly, as I released my grip on the need to control everything, I rediscovered a part of myself I thought I'd lost—a sense of curiosity and wonder that had been buried under the weight of responsibilities.

"Curiosity is the engine of achievement," Sir Ken Robinson once said, and I've found this to be profoundly true. My journey back to curiosity began with a bold decision: I left my corporate job and took an 11-month break. Those months were life-changing. I spent much of that time reading, letting myself dive into book after book. Each one opened my eyes to new ideas, teaching me things I'd never taken the time to explore before. I realised that my natural curiosity, the spark of wonder I'd felt as a child, had been stifled by the pressures of adulthood and the fear of failing. With more time to breathe and reflect, I started working on quieting my overactive mind. It was like peeling back layers of stress and routine to find that small, curious part of me again. As I slowed down, I noticed the world around me in a way I hadn't for years.

I remember walking in nature with friends, discussing dreams and laughing without restraint. Those moments felt magical, as if I was seeing the world through fresh eyes. Nature became a refuge where I could just be, free from the constant need to be productive. It felt like finding joy again, a joy I hadn't even realised was missing.

Curiosity took root in my daily life. I started journaling regularly, writing down my thoughts and paying attention to my dreams. I came across Athena Laz's *The Alchemy of Dreams*, which suggests that our dreams are like mirrors, reflecting what we might not see in ourselves. Her ideas resonated with me. My dreams, once ignored, started to guide me toward things I needed to change or embrace. Journaling about them helped me uncover patterns and deeper truths about my life. At the same time, I began noticing how my body seemed to communicate with me. I was reminded of something Bessel van der Kolk wrote in *The Body Keeps the Score*: "The body remembers what we forget." His words struck a chord. I began to see that the aches and pains I carried were often tied to emotions I hadn't dealt with. This realisation pushed me to explore healing practices like ayahuasca ceremonies, sound therapy, and deep breathing meditation. Each one opened a door to parts of myself I hadn't fully understood before. I started seeing meditation not just as a way to calm my mind, but as a tool to sit with discomfort and work through it. It felt as though my body was teaching me how to listen, gently guiding me toward healing and self-compassion.

Of course, there were moments when I sought escape instead of facing my emotions. I'd binge-watch Netflix, letting the hours slip by in an attempt to avoid my thoughts. But even in those moments, I found lessons. I also came across Marisa Peer's *Tell Yourself a Better Lie*, which talks about how our beliefs shape our lives. She writes, "Change the narrative, change your life." Her words encouraged me to shift my inner dialogue. Instead of being stuck in negative thought loops, I began replacing those thoughts with kinder, more supportive ones. This practice of reframing my beliefs became a powerful way to rebuild my confidence. As I changed the way I talked to myself, I started seeing my life in a new light. Instead of focusing on my mistakes, I began to appreciate the lessons they'd taught me. Every failure, every wrong turn, had shaped who I was becoming.

With each step, I felt more grateful. The struggles I'd faced were no longer just painful memories; they were part of a bigger story—my story. A story of growth, resilience, and transformation. I came to see that the power to change how I viewed my life was always within me. By letting go of control, I discovered a world full of possibilities.

Lynn Twist captures this beautifully in *The Soul of Money* when she says, "The quality of your life is determined by how you choose to relate to what you have." Her words helped me shift from a mindset of scarcity to one of abundance. I started seeing the world as a place full of opportunities for growth and joy, and I trusted that life had more to offer than I could have imagined. As I reflect on this journey, I feel immense compassion for the person I've become. Each challenge, each victory, has been a piece of the puzzle that makes up who I am today. Ralph Waldo Emerson once said, "What lies behind us and what lies before us are tiny matters compared to what lies within us." Those words remind me that my strength comes from within, and that inner strength has carried me through even the hardest times.

Today, I feel a deep sense of gratitude for the life I've built and the person I've grown into. I've learned to love myself in a way I never thought possible, and that self-love has opened my heart to others. I feel connected to the people and the world around me in a way that fills me with hope and joy. This journey back to curiosity has been anything but easy, but it's also been the most rewarding experience of my life. I've found my inner child again, the part of me that looks at life with wonder and excitement. And even though the road has been filled with challenges, each one has helped me grow stronger.

In Sarah Prout's words, "When you learn to be the love, you create a life that reflects the beauty of your heart." These words remind me that love is more than just a feeling—it's a way of being. As I continue to nurture this love within myself, I know it will radiate outward, transforming not just my life but the lives of those around me.

The Courage to Choose Happiness Over Comfort

Letting go of what's familiar and stepping into the unknown is often talked about like it's an exciting adventure, but the truth is, it's incredibly hard. It takes a kind of courage I didn't know I had—a willingness to face the fears that kept me stuck in a life shaped by what others expected of me. Curiosity became the light that guided me through this process, helping me see possibilities I'd never considered before. Each risk I took stirred a mix of fear and hope, challenging me to trust in something bigger than my doubts. Choosing to embrace being single wasn't just about me—it deeply impacted my children, too. It was a leap into an emotional unknown for all of us, but a small voice inside urged me to believe it could lead to stronger connections and a life that felt truer to who we are.

Leaving my corporate job was another big step into uncertainty. For years, the steady paycheck had felt like a safety net. But deep down, I knew I needed to find out what mattered most to me, and curiosity became my motivator. I started imagining a life where I could succeed on my terms instead of staying stuck in a routine that didn't fulfil me. Breaking away from what was familiar felt like shedding an old layer of skin that had grown too tight. After years of living in a predictable, stable world, choosing the unknown felt risky—not just for me but for my kids too. I worried about their education and what sacrifices we might have to make. But I also knew that staying in a life that no longer served me wasn't the answer. Curiosity gave me the strength to explore new possibilities and believe the risks might be worth it.

I learned that fear often isn't as real as it seems. It's more like a story we tell ourselves, and the more we believe it, the bigger it feels. I had to remind myself that I deserved joy and fulfilment. Curiosity helped me change my mindset so that I could see challenges as chances to grow instead of problems to avoid. I realised I didn't just want to get by—I wanted to live fully. And making that choice became something I worked at every day. Some people might say my decisions were foolish, and maybe they're right. But if being foolish means finding happiness, then I'm okay with that. I used to have everything the world says you need to be successful—status, money, and security—but none of it made me happy. I'd rather have a life filled with meaning than one full of things that don't really matter.

Now, as I stand on the edge of the unknown, I feel stronger with every step I take. Each leap reminds me that I'm capable of building a brighter future for myself. Curiosity keeps me moving forward, even when I stumble. I've learned to embrace my mistakes, value vulnerability, and trust that I'm on the right path. I don't have all the answers, but I've found peace in knowing that life is a journey. I choose to thrive, and with that choice comes self-compassion. It's a reminder that we're all finding our way, and in that shared struggle, we can find strength together.

Manifesting My Future Aspirations

Each morning, I wake up with a heart full of hope and a strong sense of purpose, dreaming of a life that truly aligns with my passions and feeds my soul. I believe deeply in the power of manifestation—the idea that by clearly imagining what I want and believing in it, I can start building the path to make it happen. Most days, this feels natural and encouraging, but there are also times when reality reminds me that reaching my dreams takes hard work and a willingness to adapt. Sometimes, the challenges of the world make it hard to hold on to my vision. As a parent, I feel a deep responsibility to provide the best opportunities for my children. That responsibility can feel heavy, tying me to a corporate world that doesn't always match my true passions.

Even so, I stay motivated by looking at what I've already achieved through manifestation. For the past four years, I've focused on a vision of freedom, guided by the mantra "Freedom to Shine." I've worked hard to reach this point in my life, and I'm proud to say I've broken free from the limits that used to hold me back. Now, I'm ready to embrace all the opportunities that life has to offer.

Living in a world driven by capitalism can often feel overwhelming, especially when the pursuit of a living seems to overshadow my dreams. However, I am determined to find a way to balance my passions with the practical need to earn money. I envision a future where I work on meaningful projects in human resources, helping organisations navigate change while managing the complexities of office dynamics.

I imagine a world where I can positively impact individuals, guiding them to live more consciously and in harmony with others. I aspire to support those going through transformative moments in their lives, helping them find clarity and purpose. At the same time, I want to assist those who must navigate the corporate landscape, enabling them to maintain a healthy balance and stay true to their authentic selves, even amidst the mindless games and politics that often permeate the workplace. My goal is to empower these individuals to thrive in a system that, while necessary, can sometimes feel stifling. By fostering a sense of community and understanding, I hope to create an environment where everyone can flourish, allowing us all to contribute to a society that values both financial stability and personal fulfilment.

I also dream of a time when my children are on their own paths, free from the financial burdens of education. In this vision of the future, I see myself living in a peaceful place—maybe the serene landscapes of Switzerland, the historical charm of the UK, or the warm, familiar surroundings of South Africa, where my roots are. My home will be modest but welcoming, nestled in nature, and open to guests seeking rest and healing. My home and business will co-exist; it won't be a large business but an intimate and cosy home where every visitor feels truly cared for. Each stay will be tailored to their needs, offering a chance for them to reconnect with themselves. I picture myself in a warm kitchen, the air filled with the aroma of fresh, plant-based meals made from local ingredients. My guests will come from all walks of life, each on their own journey, but united by a desire to grow and transform. I want to create a place that encourages stillness, where the calm of nature inspires reflection and personal breakthroughs. As a coach, I want to help people find their inner strength and realise that true fulfilment comes from within, discovered through self-reflection and personal exploration.

I imagine intimate conversations by the fire, sharing the lessons I've learned from my own journey—lessons shaped by both struggles and successes. I want to inspire others to carve their own paths instead of conforming to societal norms. I want to show that real success comes from embracing what feels true to you and using your experiences as a guide. As Ralph Waldo Emerson said, "The only person you are destined to become is the person you decide to be."

In this special home, I plan to bring together nutritionists, yoga teachers, meditation guides, and spiritual healers to create a supportive community. Together, we'll help guests care for their minds, bodies, and spirits. This vision is built on connection and compassion—a life where every moment brings me closer to fulfilment and helps others thrive. I want to leave a legacy of empowerment, encouraging others to chase their dreams and embrace their authentic selves, creating a world where everyone has the chance to flourish.

I dream of a life where my world and my work are fully in harmony. In this home, I see myself living with my two British Shorthair cats, Simba and Lena, who have brought so much love into my life since August 2023. My sons will visit occasionally, filling the house with energy and joy. I also imagine friends and family gathering here, sharing laughter and good times. I dream about finding true love with a partner; I trust that it will happen naturally, adding to the happiness in my life when the time is right.

When I think about my future, I also reflect on how far I've come in changing my relationship with money. For a long time, I lived with a scarcity mindset, always feeling like there wasn't enough—whether it was money, time, or resources. That way of thinking held me back and made me feel trapped. Over time, I've shifted to an abundance mindset, completely changing my outlook. This new perspective has opened doors I didn't know existed and helped me see possibilities where there were none before. It's given me hope and the courage to embrace life with open arms.

Through my pro bono coaching, I've been blessed to witness how even the smallest acts of generosity can create ripples of positivity that stretch far beyond what we can see. I dedicate a portion of my time—time I could have spent earning money—to offer coaching to others. This decision has been both purposeful and rewarding. Through this work, I've seen how small gestures can make a big difference in people's lives. I've had the chance to help those feeling stuck or lost in the corporate world, and in doing so, I've discovered a deeper sense of purpose within myself. Seeing others grow, rediscover their strengths, and reconnect with who they are brings me immense joy. It feels like a gift to create a space where people can thrive. To ensure my spending aligns with my values, I embrace the practice of conscious spending.

Instead of shopping mindlessly at big stores, I make an effort to support local businesses and ethical brands. I like to ask questions about how products are made and where they come from. I still remember how happy I felt when I bought a beautiful handwoven basket from a fair-trade shop. Knowing that the money went directly to artisans who were paid fairly made the purchase even more special. That small act connected me to a bigger community and reminded me that every franc I spend is like casting a vote for the kind of world I want to help create. My unwavering support for Indigenous wisdom and the protection of our planet will remain a cornerstone of my future. This commitment is about more than just my personal journey—it's a shared responsibility to care for our planet and its people. I believe in the strength of collective action, and I'm passionate about inspiring others to participate in this important work.

As I continue down this path, I find joy in knowing that my choices can lead to meaningful contributions in an unequal world. Lynn Twist said it perfectly: "The way we spend our money reflects our values." By adopting an abundance mindset, spending consciously, and contributing collectively, I feel more connected and empowered than ever before. I'm deeply thankful for the chance to use my resources to make a positive impact and invite others to join me on this shared journey. Together, we can create a ripple effect of hope and empowerment, ensuring that our dreams lift not just us, but also those around us.

In this expansive, longer-term vision, I see a life where my actions create a legacy of compassion, connection, and empowerment. I want to be a source of encouragement for others, showing them that our dreams can work together to build a better world. Every step I take is rooted in love and intention, reflecting my belief that when we support one another, we can create a future filled with hope and opportunity. With each endeavour, I am committed to fostering a sense of community and belonging. I want to create safe and welcoming spaces where people can be open about their struggles, share their stories, and explore ways to grow and heal. In these spaces, we'll support one another in embracing authenticity and courage, reminding ourselves that our challenges can make us stronger.

My Journey Towards The Change Canvas

With my long-term vision visually represented on my vision board, I have begun taking meaningful steps toward it, each action generating the energy needed to bring that vision to life. I am determined to make choices that allow me to live as my true self. In this context, I have finally decided to let go of the security of the corporate world and take the risk of establishing my own small business, which will enable me to leverage my experiences in serving corporate clients and individuals seeking transformation. When I began writing my book, I experienced a surge of inspiration that prompted a significant shift in my life. I've always felt a thrill in uniting diverse voices and perspectives, believing in the power of storytelling to break down barriers and build bridges. This fosters a more inclusive world where every voice is valued. With this renewed inspiration, I boldly embarked on a new adventure: creating my own boutique business. This was my chance to focus on what truly excites me.

At The Change Canvas, I envision guiding individuals and organisations on their journeys of self-discovery. My purpose is clear: to empower people to express their inner truth and vision, helping them craft a more authentic life. Through tailored coaching and consulting, I aim to ignite the transformative power of conscious leadership, personal growth, and meaningful connections. I am committed to fostering an environment of empathy and support, one that resonates with each person's unique experiences.

What is The Change Canvas?

Drawing from my own experiences, I wish to guide people through the complexities of life. Societal pressures often force us to wear different masks, but through The Change Canvas, I aim to help individuals challenge these norms. My struggles with self-discovery inspired me to write "Awakening to Wholeness: A Life Unmasked," where I share my transformative journey and emphasise the importance of living authentically.

I focus on conscious living and leadership, helping everyone thrive through compassion. I envision workshops that create a culture of openness and trust, where participants learn to lead with their true selves. I believe that when leaders embrace their unique identities, they inspire those around them, fostering a collaborative environment where everyone can contribute.

Transformational retreats will invite participants on journeys of introspection, empowering them to reconnect with their truest selves and find lasting joy. I also aspire to offer personalised career development programmes, helping individuals align their professional paths with their values.

At The Change Canvas, I aim to create workplaces rooted in respect and inclusivity. With my multicultural background, I understand the importance of fostering a culture of understanding and collaboration. I hope to work with organisations to navigate change effectively, crafting tailored strategies that empower them to drive change independently.

Ultimately, The Change Canvas is about building a community. I invite clients to embark on a journey of self-discovery and creation, celebrating the rich tapestry of experiences that bind us together.

In conclusion

As I look ahead, I remain steadfast in my commitment to this vision. I believe that together, we can illuminate the path toward a brighter future. Each small action I take stands as a testament to the transformative power of our collective dreams, inspiring us to reshape not only our lives but also the world around us.

I invite you to join me on this journey of authenticity and self-discovery. Together, we can weave a rich tapestry of shared experiences where each voice contributes to a harmonious symphony of growth and healing. Your story matters deeply; it holds the potential to spark change and inspire others. Together, we can cultivate a vibrant community that uplifts, empowers, and embraces each individual's unique journey. Let us step boldly into the unknown, igniting the light within us all. As we share our truths and support one another, we create a sanctuary where resilience flourishes and hope prevails. In this space, we transform our vulnerabilities into strengths, forging connections that uplift and inspire.

In the heart of transformation, a powerful legacy awaits us—one that encourages every seeker to embrace their authenticity and step into their brilliance. Together, we can manifest a future that reflects our dreams and brings forth a wave of positive change that resonates far beyond ourselves. Let us embark on this journey not just as individuals but as a united force ready to embrace the light and share it with the world.

EPILOGUE: ANSWERING THE QUESTION: WHO AM I?

As I sit and reflect on the journey I've shared in these pages, I hope you, dear reader, can see the threads that run through my story—threads of struggle, resilience, and, most importantly, transformation. Back in 2019, my life was a whirlwind of roles: Vice President of Human Resources, wife, mother, sister, aunt, dual citizen. I carried these titles like shields, believing they defined who I was and gave me value. But behind the weight of these labels, I wrestled with an emptiness I couldn't shake—a longing for something real, something truly me.

Amid the hustle of everyday life, I often felt like an actor in a play, wearing different masks to meet everyone's expectations. Each role brought its own demands, making me feel like I was building a wall that hid who I really was. The opening of my book reflects this reality, touching on the heavy armour we wear to protect ourselves from the world's pressures. It sets the tone for a deeper exploration of how these roles can fragment us, leaving us disconnected from our true selves.

At the heart of my reflections is the idea of identity—something constantly shaped by our families, cultures, and the society we live in. I look at how these outside forces shaped me and how I struggled to break free from them in my search for authenticity. My upbringing and societal expectations often felt like chains, pulling me in directions that weren't always true to who I was. This part of my story is about untangling those threads and learning to see myself more clearly.

My journey toward clarity—driven by self-reflection and therapy—marks a turning point in my life. It wasn't a quick or easy process. It meant facing hard truths and coming to terms with the parts of my past I wanted to ignore. But through it all, I learned to embrace vulnerability and to accept my flaws as an essential part of who I am. This shift from confusion to understanding is one of the most important themes in my story.

Love also played a big role in my reflections. Love has a dual nature—it can lift us up, but it can also hold us down. In this book, I've explored how love has shaped my journey, from moments of pure joy and connection to times of pain and doubt. These experiences taught me about the power of love to shape our understanding of ourselves and our place in the world.

This epilogue isn't just an ending; it's a way of tying together the lessons I've learned and the questions I've grappled with. "Who am I?" is a question that doesn't have one answer. It's a journey—a process of discovery that continues with every step I take.

My healing journey, marked by deep self-reflection and facing old wounds, has been at the heart of my transformation. I learned the importance of letting go of the past to fully live in the present. This journey included exploring ancient wisdom through spiritual practices like ayahuasca ceremonies and sound medicine meditations. These experiences opened my mind and heart, helping me see beyond the limits of my everyday life and connect with deeper parts of myself and the universe.

Finding freedom in authenticity came from reclaiming my sense of self. I discovered the joy and strength that come from embracing who I truly am. I realised that being authentic isn't just about dropping the masks we wear; it's a choice to live in a way that reflects our values and beliefs. The question, "Who am I?" lies at the core of this book. It's an invitation for readers to start their own journey of self-discovery, to look past the layers of societal expectations and uncover their true selves.

By sharing my story, I hope to help others who may be facing similar challenges. The journey of discovering who you are isn't a straight road; it's full of twists and turns, with moments of joy and clarity mixed with times of doubt and confusion. But it's through this messy, beautiful process that we find our true voice and reclaim control over our own story. I invite you to join me in this exploration—to think about your own identity and embrace the complexities of being human. Together, we can move toward a life of authenticity and wholeness.

As I share my experiences, I encourage you to consider one fundamental question: "Who am I?" That question sparked my awakening, and I hope it will inspire you as well. Through the wisdom of Michael Singer's *The Untethered Soul*, I learned how powerful self-reflection can be. I also learned that true freedom comes from letting go of society's expectations and stepping back to observe life as it unfolds without judgment.

The journey to discovering yourself isn't straightforward. It can be painful and confusing, with moments of insight and times when nothing makes sense. Therapy was a crucial part of my journey, helping me see myself more clearly, even though it didn't always bring the relief I was seeking. It was only when I allowed myself to dig deeper—connecting my conscious and subconscious thoughts—that I started to take back my story. This kind of healing requires courage and vulnerability, but it's worth it.

Throughout my book, the paradox of love has been a guiding theme. Love can be a source of comfort and healing, but it can also feel stifling at times. As you read my story, I hope it helps you reflect on your own relationships and see both the light and the dark within them. True growth often comes from facing both sides of love—the nurturing and the challenging—and finding a balance between them.

One of the biggest lessons I've learned is the importance of embracing uncertainty. The future, which once filled me with anxiety, has become a canvas of endless possibilities. I've learned to trust life as it unfolds, to go with its flow rather than fight against it. If there's one message I want you to take away, it's this: It's okay not to have all the answers. Embrace the unknown and let it guide you to new opportunities and discoveries.

As I bring this book to a close, I feel overwhelming gratitude—for the struggles that shaped me, for the love that helped me heal, and for the lessons I've learned along the way. I hope my story speaks to you and inspires you to start your own journey of self-discovery. Remember, you are more than your circumstances or the roles you play. You are the observer of your own life, capable of finding peace and wholeness in its complexities.

So, who are you? I invite you to explore that question with an open heart and mind. Trust that, like me, you will uncover the beauty and strength of simply being yourself. Embrace the journey, because that's where you'll find your true self.

ACKNOWLEDGEMENTS

In quiet moments of reflection, I am filled with gratitude and a deep love for my twin boys. You are the shining lights in my life, guiding me through the darkness I once faced. This book is more than just a collection of my thoughts; it is a journey—a story stitched together with experiences of joy, pain, struggle, and growth.

This book is my promise to you, my dear sons. It is my way of sharing the ups and downs of my life—a journey of discovering myself and turning the shadows of my past into something brighter. Through these pages, I hope to show you the challenges that shaped me and the moments that kept me going when I thought I couldn't.

As I look back, I realise how many people have left their mark on my life. To my sister, Dawn, your constant love and support have been a safe haven for me. You've reminded me, time and time again, that family is the anchor in life's stormy seas. Your belief in me has given me the strength to keep going. To my nieces, Melanie and Rozanne: Melanie, your passion for books has inspired me to grow in ways I never thought was possible. Rozanne, your courage and kindness in tough times have shown me how to face challenges with love and generosity.

To Nicole, my cherished friend and mentor, thank you for guiding me and helping me see possibilities I had forgotten. Your faith in me, even when I doubted myself, has encouraged me to dig deeper and embrace who I truly am. You've taught me how powerful it is to be vulnerable and to share our stories.

To Bonita, Emily, Christine, and Emma, your unwavering presence has been my rock during my hardest days. You've listened without judgment, shared your wisdom with care, and reminded me that I am never truly alone. Your friendship proves the strength of sisterhood and the healing power of connection.

Finally, to my ex-husband, thank you. We spent 25 years knowing each other, 19 of them as husband and wife. Our time together, though filled with its share of highs and lows, has deeply influenced who I am today. I recognise how our shared journey taught me lessons and brought me to a greater understanding of myself. The challenges we faced together played a part in igniting my path toward self-awareness, and for that, I will always be grateful. Thank you for being part of that chapter in my life.

To everyone mentioned here, thank you for believing in me when I struggled to believe in myself and for encouraging me to share my story. This book belongs as much to you as it does to me. It celebrates the love, resilience, and connection that have guided me to be braver.

And to my precious sons, I hope that when you read this book, you'll understand why I made the difficult decision to part ways with your father. It was a choice made with love—love for myself and love for you. It wasn't easy, but it was necessary. I want you to know that finding happiness and living authentically is possible, even when the journey is uncertain. You are my greatest inspiration, and my wish is for you to grow up knowing that true strength comes from being true to yourself.

REFERENCES

All poems began with the author's original words, which were then refined and shaped with the assistance of Ask AI, an AI language model by Codeway. This collaborative process ensured that the final pieces authentically conveyed the story the author aimed to unfold in each chapter.

1. **Prologue: Life and a Dance of Roles**

- Singer, Michael A. (2007). *The Untethered Soul: The Journey Beyond Yourself.* New Harbinger Publications.
- Brach, Tara. (2019). *Radical Compassion: Learning to Love Yourself Through the Practice of Forgiveness*. Bantam.
- Perry, B. & Winfrey, O. (2021). *"What Happened to You?: Conversations on Trauma, Resilience, and Healing".* Flatiron Books.
- Brach, Tara. (2021) *"Radical Compassion: Learning to Love Yourself and Your World with the Practice of R.A.I.N."* HarperOne.
- Kaur, Rupi. (2017) *"The Sun and Her Flowers."* Andrews McMeel Publishing.

2. **How Lineage and Society Shape Our Identity**

a) **Moving Forward with Gratitude: Honouring our Roots**

- Lewey, V. (2002). *Thunder from a clear sky: A true South African story.*

b) **Forging Resilience: A Silent Defence for the Heart**

- Singer, Michael A. (2007) The Untethered Soul: The Journey Beyond Yourself. New Harbinger Publications.

- Winfrey, Oprah, and Dr. Bruce Perry. (2021) What Happened to You? Flatiron Books.
- Brown, Brené. (2010) The gifts of imperfection: Let go of who you think you're supposed to be and embrace who you are. Hazelden Publishing.
- Prout, Sarah. (2022) Be the Love: Seven Ways to Unlock Your Heart and Manifest Happiness. St Martins Essentials.
- Brown, Brené. (2018) Dare to Lead: Brave Work. Tough Conversations. Whole Hearts. Penguin Press.
- Brown, Brené. (2012) Daring Greatly: How the Courage to Be Vulnerable Transforms the Way We Live, Love, Parent, and Lead. Gotham Books.
- Brown, Brené. (2017) Braving the Wilderness: The Quest for True Belonging and the Courage to Stand Alone. Spiegel & Grau.
- Covey, Stephen. R. (1989) The seven habits of highly effective people: Powerful lessons in personal change. Simon & Schuster.
- Fulghum, Robert. (1986) All I Really Need to Know I Learned in Kindergarten: Uncommon Thoughts on Common Things. New York: Villard Books.
- Angelou, Maya. (1981) The Heart of a Woman. Random House.

3. The Turning Point: Awakening Through Awareness

a) Crossing the Threshold: Closing a Chapter

- Gilbert, E. (2006). Eat, Pray, Love: One Woman's Search for Everything Across Italy, India and Indonesia. New York: Viking Penguin.

b) Truths Unveiled: Confronting the Dark Heart of Deception

- Reference: Angelou, M. (1993). "Wouldn't Take Nothing for My Journey Now". Random House.

c) From Corporate Shadows to Clarity: Breaking Free

- Whitworth, L., Kimsey-House, H., Kimsey-House, K., & Sandahl, P. (2010). "Co-Active Coaching: Changing Business, Transforming Lives". 2nd ed. Nicholas Brealey Publishing.
- Brown, Brené. (2018) "Dare to Lead: Brave Work. Tough Conversations." Whole Hearts.
- Grant, Adam. (2021) "Think Again: The Power of Knowing What You Don't Know.
- Singer, Michael A. (2007) The Untethered Soul: The Journey Beyond Yourself. New Harbinger Publications.

4. Love's Complexity: From Attachment to Acceptance

- Prout, Sarah. (2022) Be the Love: Seven Ways to Unlock Your Heart and Manifest Happiness. St Martins Essentials.

a) Love as a Partner: Embracing the Journey of Marriage

- The Poem "What is Love" was generated fully by Ask AI, an AI language model by Codeway.
- Leadership Circle. (n.d.). Leadership Circle Profile 360 feedback.
- Chapman, Gary. (1992). The 5 Love Languages: How to Express Heartfelt Commitment to Your Family. Northfield Publishing.
- Durvasula, R. (2020). "Should I Stay or Should I Go?: Surviving a Relationship with a Narcissist". New Harbinger Publications.
- Martinez-Lewi, L. (2015). "Freeing Yourself from the Narcissist in Your Life". Health Communications, Inc.

b) Love as a Mother: Nurturing Bonds and Unconditional Connection

- Connections in Mind. (n.d.). Executive functioning parents coaching program. Retrieved 22 October 2024, from https://www.connectionsinmind.co.uk

c) Love Among Family and Friends: The Strength of Cherished Connections

- Quindlen, Anna. (2000). A Short Guide to a Happy Life. Random House.
- Heimann, Nicole. (2016). How to Develop the Authentic Leader in You.
- Angelou, Maya. (2013) Mom & Me & Mom. Random House.

d) Nourishing Love: Cultivating a Relationship with What I Feed My Body

- Chapman, Gary. (1992). The 5 Love Languages: How to Express Heartfelt Commitment to Your Family. Northfield Publishing.
- Gay, Roxanne. (2017). Hunger: A Memoir of (My) Body. HarperCollins.
- Fuhrman, Joel. (2003) Eat to Live: The Amazing Nutrient-Rich Program for Fast and Sustained Weight Loss. HarperCollins.
- Prout, Sarah. (2022) Be the Love: Seven Ways to Unlock Your Heart and Manifest Happiness. St Martins Essentials.

5. Spiritual Healing: Releasing the Wounds of the Past

- Tolle, E. (2005). A new earth: Awakening to your life's purpose. Penguin Group.
- Manari Ushigua, Political and Spiritual Leader of the Sàpara Nation in Ecuadorian Amazon
- Dr. Arne Heissel, modern mystic, energy healer and visionary in global health
- Thompson, J. (2001). The Healing Power of Sound: Recovery from Life-Threatening Illness Using Sound, Music, and Vibration. New York: Healing Arts Press.

6. Freedom Found: Embracing Authenticity

a) Beyond Myself: Discovering the Wholeness Within

- Singer, Michael A (2007). *The Untethered Soul: The Journey Beyond Yourself.* New Harbinger Publications.
- Shepherd, Philip. (2019) "Radical Wholeness: The Embodied Present and the Ordinary Grace of Being". North Atlantic Books.
- Perry, B. & Winfrey, O. (2021). "*What Happened to You?: Conversations on Trauma, Resilience, and Healing*". Flatiron Books.
- Brown, Brené. (2012) *Daring Greatly: How the Courage to Be Vulnerable Transforms the Way We Live, Love, Parent, and Lead.* Gotham Books
- Gilbert, E. (2006). *Eat, Pray, Love: One Woman's Search for Everything Across Italy, India and Indonesia.* New York: Viking Penguin.
- Peers, Marisa. (2019) *I Am Enough: Mark Your Path to Self-Love and Acceptance.* Hay House.
- Mandela, Nelson. "As we let our own lights shine, we unconsciously give others the permission to do the same."

b) Embracing the Unknown: Welcoming Future Possibilities

- Singer, Michael A (2007). *The Untethered Soul: The Journey Beyond Yourself.* New Harbinger Publications.

- Tolle, Eckhart. (1999) *The Power of Now: A Guide to Spiritual Enlightenment.* New World Library.
- Robinson, Ken. (2011) "Out of Our Minds: Learning to be Creative". Capstone.
- Twist, Lynn. (2017) "The Soul of Money: Transforming Your Relationship with Money and Life". Norton.
- Emerson, Ralph Waldo. (1841) "Self-Reliance".
- Prout, Sarah. (2022) *Be the Love: Seven Ways to Unlock Your Heart and Manifest Happiness.* St Martins Essentials.
- van der Kolk, B. (2014). "The Body Keeps the Score: Brain, Mind, and Body in the Healing of Trauma". Viking.
- Peer, M. (2018). "Tell Yourself a Better Lie: Use the Power of Your Mind to Change Your Life". HarperCollins.
- Laz, A. (2021). *The alchemy of your dreams. A Modern Guide to the Ancient Art of Lucid Dreaming and Interpretation.* Penguin Publishing Group
- Emerson, R. W. (n.d.). "The only person you are destined to become is the person you decide to be."

7. Epilogue: Answering the Question: Who am I?

- Singer, Michael A. (2007) *The Untethered Soul: The Journey Beyond Yourself.* New Harbinger Publications.

Bios for Spiritual Healing: Releasing the Wounds of the Past

Manari Ushigua is a traditional healer and leader of the Sàpara Nation in the Ecuadorian Amazon. The Sàpara Nation is recognised by UNESCO as an Intangible Cultural Heritage of Humanity. Manari has been a key figure in the Indigenous movement of Ecuador as the Vice President of CONAIE (The National Indigenous Organization of Ecuador) from 2013-2016, and as the President of the Sàpara Indigenous Federation from 1999 to 2012. Manari has participated in international events, like the COP21 UN Climate Summit and the UN Universal Periodic Review of Human Rights, raising awareness about the threat to his homeland. As a defender of Indigenous rights, he has managed to conserve more than 276,000 hectares of primary forest threatened by extractive industries. Manari is the co-founder of the

Naku Center, creating a new economic model in the Amazon that is based around cultural and forest preservation.

Arne Heissel, PhD

Following a 25+ years global leadership career in the established healthcare system, Dr. Arne turned the altered state of consciousness expert, modern mystic and energy healer. He developed his own healing method. In 2022, he founded his company, Human Intelligence Academy, and is currently in the early launch phase of his new pioneering program for holistic healing, peak performance and personal transformation program, Transcend21: The Consciousness Codex. The Gateway to Healing, Peak Performance, and Transcendence". This program combines cutting-edge science, intuitive insights, deep meditation and ancient wisdom like no other, offering a unique pathway to awaken the inner healer for physical, emotional and spiritual healing, peak performance and transcendence. His programs, transformative workshops, retreats and energy sessions empower clients on their journeys towards greater awareness, fulfilment, resilience in times of adversity, intuition and inner peace. Offerings are in person or online in English or German language. For more information about his services and approach, visit www.quantumandheart,www.codex21,www.humanintelligenceacademy or WhatsApp at +491793665909